American Sign Language
for Beginners

Jacob Vinson

COPYRIGHT

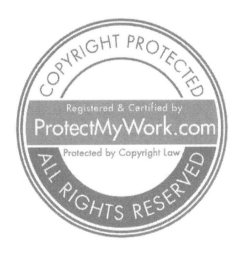

Table of Contents

The mission

This book is for those eager to learn ASL, whether for family, work, or community engagement. Basic ASL knowledge improves communication and can make a difference in emergency situations. Furthermore, it promotes the rights of the deaf community, which still needs support to achieve the recognition it deserves.

This book serves as a valuable resource designed to provide beginners with the fundamentals of all aspects of ASL in the most inclusive way. Through the accompanying videos and practical exercises, you'll have the opportunity to continually practice and advance to higher proficiency levels.

The division into three books will allow you to grow gradually and engage in your first conversations within just a few days:

Book 1 covers all the ASL basics.
Book 2 focuses on greetings and practical communication.
Book 3 will guide you in mastering tenses and verb conjugations.

Before embarking on your journey to learn American Sign Language (ASL) through the pages of this book, let me offer you a glimpse into the passion and dedication of someone who played a crucial role in bringing this project to life.

Allow me to introduce Daisy, a remarkable individual whose commitment to ASL goes beyond the ordinary. She isn't deaf, nor does she have any deaf family members. You might wonder, why did she choose to learn and teach ASL? Let me share her inspiring words:

"I learned ASL to better connect with deaf individuals, not relying on interpreters or text messages, but to demonstrate that I care enough to communicate with them in the language of their hearts. I don't have any deaf individuals in my family, but I've witnessed the struggles of deaf people trying to convey basic thoughts; they are often ignored or treated disrespectfully. Nevertheless, I am always thrilled to bridge the communication gap by serving as their voice and ears. Together, we can all contribute to making the world a more inclusive place for millions of deaf individuals worldwide."

BOOK 1:

ASL Essentials

Go to the last page and scan the QR code to access an entire collection of bonus tutorial videos.

American Sign Language origins:

ASL is a visual language, complete with grammar, based on specific hand gestures, body movements and facial expressions and does not necessarily reflect English words.

It has a long history, and its journey to existence was challenging.
For the first time, in the 1700s, Charles-Michel de l'Épée, known as the Father of the Deaf, created an educational method for others to learn sign language.

In 1817 an American educator named Thomas Hopkins Gallaudet, along with a French teacher named Laurent Clerc and an American physician named Mason Cogswell, co-founded the first permanent institution for the education of the deaf in North America, and he became its first principal. When it was first opened it was called "The Connecticut Asylum for the Education and Instruction of Deaf and Dumb Persons". The school was subsequently renamed "The American School for the Deaf (ASD)" and in 1821 moved to 139 Main Street, West Hartford. The school remains the oldest existing school for the deaf in North America.
However, the ASL was officially recognized just in 1960.
So, ASL originates from France, and that's why it is very similar to French Sign Language and quite different from British Sign Language
American Sign Language is predominantly used in the United States and in many parts of Canada, so it is not a universal language, indeed there are lots of "slang" movements and slight regional distinctions and this book does its best to represent the most common form of each sign.

Anyway, behind English, Spanish and Chinese, ASL is the fourth most widely used language in the US with around 2 million users.

Define the signing size:

Whenever you're signing you need to make sure that your sign occupies the right amount of space.

Some signs go above the head but typically you're going to keep them in a space between your head and your low chest.

So, don't sign really small and don't sign really big.

Besides, I always recommend practicing in the mirror so you can check how your signs look like managing to improve them.

Which hand do I use?

Look at which is your dominant hand, that's the hand you're going to be using consistently to avoid confusion.

For instance, if you are right-handed, whenever you're signing use your right hand for the main part of the sign and your non-dominant hand for the supportive part.

Once you have chosen which is your dominant hand try to be always consistent, and avoid switching the role of your hands.

The Five Parameters:

Each sign you'll learn has five parameters that you need to pay close attention to as you go through the book. The five parameters are:

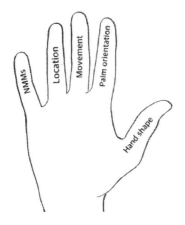

1. Hand shape
2. Palm orientation
3. Movement
4. Location
5. Non-manual markers (NMMs)

1. Hand shape

Each sign is composed of one, two, or more hand shapes. This is the shape that your hand is in to form a sign. <u>If you change the hand shape of a sign, you can alter the meaning significantly.</u>

Here there are the most common hand shapes you'll see:

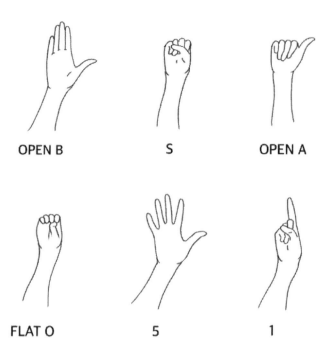

OPEN B   S   OPEN A

FLAT O   5   1

And now, I want to show you an example in which you can understand the importance of this parameter. In the first case you use a "1" handshape instead in the second case you use a "open B" handshape.

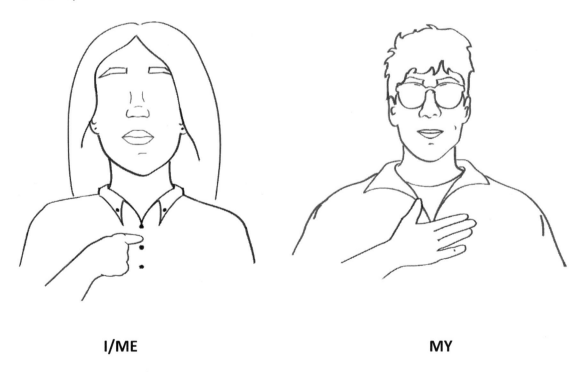

I/ME   MY

2. Palm orientation

Palm orientation means the direction your palm is facing. Your palm can be up, down, to the side, facing your body, or at a specific angle. Sometimes a sign can start with one palm orientation and move into another. Be aware of these changes.

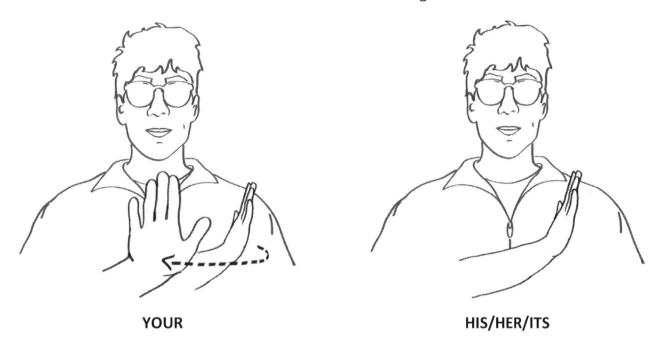

YOUR   HIS/HER/ITS

3. Movement

There are multiple types of movements you can make signing. Sometimes you may need to tap, twist, make a circle, shake, or a combination of any of these movements. Movement is a big part of what makes signing so much fun.

For instance, "to fly" is signed like "airplane" but with added forward motion.

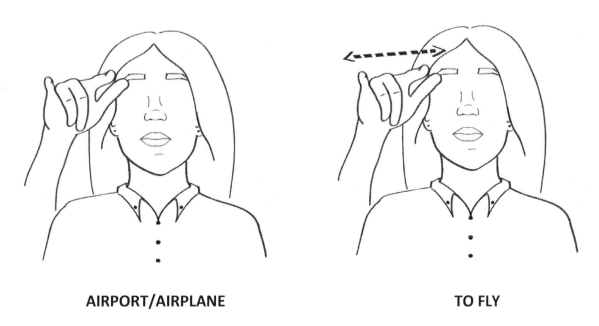

AIRPORT/AIRPLANE   TO FLY

4. Location

Every sign has a specific location. For instance, you sign MOM pointing your thumb at your chin and you sign DAD pointing it at your forehead. As you can see, everything (hand shape, palm orientation, etc.) is the same except for the location.

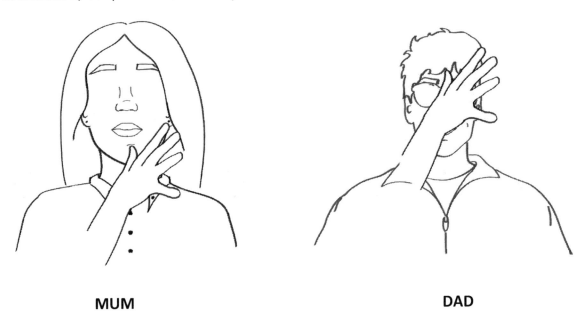

MUM   DAD

5. Non-manual markers - NMMs (facial expression)

This is everything to do with your facial expression and body language.

Think of them as the inflection in your voice and the punctuation in your writing. Without inflection in our voices, it would be difficult to determine the true meaning of what someone says to us. Facial expressions are to ASL as punctuation is to the written word.

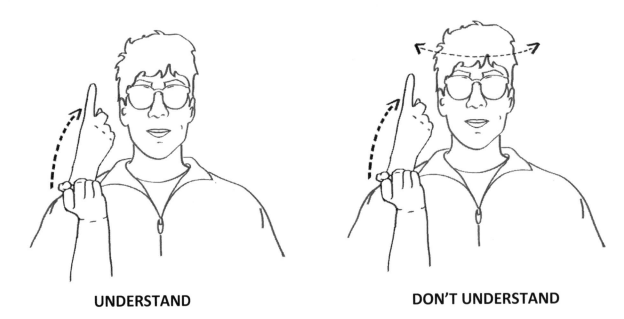

UNDERSTAND   DON'T UNDERSTAND

ASL negation and affirmation

As we have just seen in the last example, negative sentences are made just adding a facial expression. Here below you can learn the most used words:

- To say "**YES**", take a hand and make it into a fist and bob it back and forth, resembling a head nodding. To sign "**OK**" simply sign the ASL letters "O" and "K" successively.

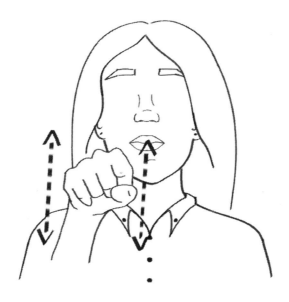

YES

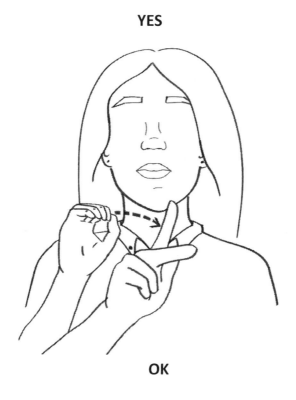

OK

- To sign "**NO**", simply take your index finger, middle finger and thumb and closed them together. To sign "**NOT**", create an "A" hand shape with the thumb extending slightly more than usual. Position the thumb under your chin and swiftly move your hand a few inches forward. <u>Typically, accompany this sign with a negative headshake.</u>

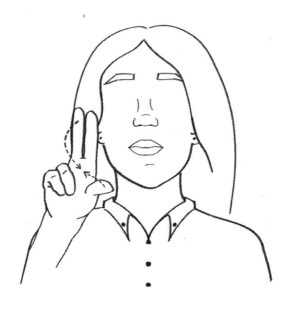

NO

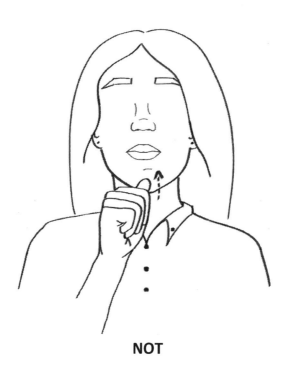

NOT

Fingerspelling

There is an ASL unique sign for each letter of the alphabet.
Fingerspelling is the use of the signed alphabet to spell words and it's quite common in ASL.
Fingerspelling is used to:

- Spell people's names or other proper nouns, such as places, titles, or organization names that do not have a designated ASL sign.
- Spell words from spoken language that don't have a designated sign, such as slang or profession-specific jargon.
- Spell words that you do not know the ASL sign for.
- Some people prefer to fingerspell even if there is an ASL sign for a word. There is nothing wrong with that, fingerspelling can be used as often as one would like.

Fingerspelling takes practice. You need to learn the signs that make up the alphabet and you need to learn to string the signs together to make words.

Here a summary of the main rules for fingerspelling:

- Hold your hand upright at approximately shoulder height;
- Keep your hand stable, avoiding any up-and-down bouncing or back-and-forth movements;
- <u>Accuracy is always better then speed</u>;
- Maintain a forward palm orientation (with the exception of the letters G and H);
- When you fingerspell a whole word, avoid to pronounce every single letter, instead say the whole word;
- Introduce a brief pause between each word when fingerspelling multiple words;
- *For words containing double letters, slid your hand to the side or pulls it to emphasize the repeated letter.

Alphabet

Similar to traditional English, American Sign Language (ASL) follows a standard set of 26 alphabets and 10 numbers to facilitate learning and mastery of lessons for students.
Just like the alphabet ASL incorporates unique sign languages specifically designed to represent numerical quantities.

In the image below, you will see how to form the letters of the alphabet.

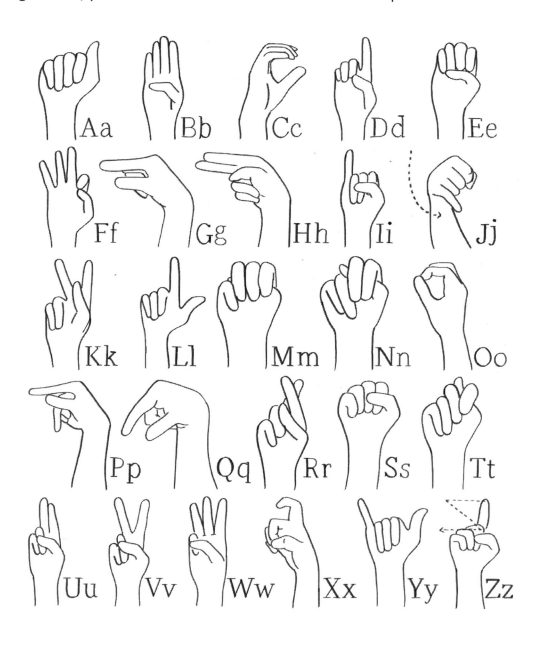

<u>Pay attention: the letters J and Z require movement, while the rest are static.</u>

A: is represented by a closed fist with your thumb placed to the side.

B: place your open palm facing forward, tuck your thumb into it, and keep the other four fingers standing upright.

C: It just looks like the shape of a letter C.

D: Your index finger is pointing up, and all other fingers are making a circle.

E: make sure your fingers are resting right on top of your thumb.

F: you have three fingers up and your index and your thumb are making a small circle. Keep the palm open and facing forward.

G: your index finger and thumb are pointed to your non-dominant side and your palm should be facing you.

H: Your index finger and your middle finger are pointed to your non-dominant side while you keep a fisted position with the other fingers.

I: Your pinky finger is pointed straight up while you keep a fisted position with the palm facing out.

*J: From the "I" position, make the shape of the letter "J" changing the palm orientation during the movement.

K: With the palm facing out, put your index and middle fingers together pointing up, split them apart and put your thumb in between.

L: From your open palm facing out, make the shape of the capital letter with your thumb and index finger.

M: From your fisted position with the thumb and pinkie closed, use your other three fingers for making the three bumps of the cursive letter "m".

N: Unlike the letter "M", use only your index and middle fingers to imitate the cursive letter "n".

O: Use the thumb to make a circle with your other fingers.

P: From your fisted position, point your index finger forward and your middle finger down, and put the tip of your thumb between them.

Q: It's just a "G" pointed downwards.

R: Your index and middle fingers are crossed with the palm facing out.

S: Form your fist and put your thumb in very front (not to the side).

T: Make your fist with the palm facing out, and put your thumb in between your index and your middle finger.

U: Put your index and middle finger together and point them up with the palm facing out.

V: It's just a "U" with the two fingers splitted.

W: It looks like the letter "W" made with your index, middle and ring fingers. Keep your palm facing out.

X: Make a Fist and raise your index finger imitating a semi hook, with the palm facing out.

Y: Your thumb and your pinkie extend outward, forming the shape of the letter Y."

*Z: Form a fist and make the shape of the Z in the air with your index finger up.

<u>Go at the end of the book and scan the QR code for watching the related video!</u>

<u>Train yourself and fingerspell all the alphabet forward and backward.</u>
<u>Practice this exercise every day and you'll be able soon to complete it in a half minute!</u>

Numbers

ASL numbers are all done with your dominant hand. Some of them can seem strange and confusing when you first learn them because the signs represent a completely new way of thinking of numbers. So, don't panic and let's start!

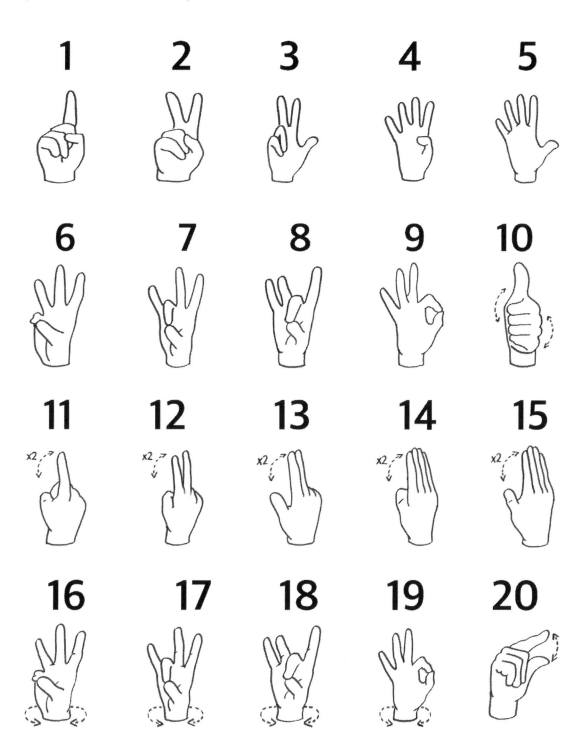

1 to 5

Numbers 1 to 5, when signed in isolation, <u>are signed with the palm facing you</u>.
You just need to imitate the picture below.

<u>Pay attention</u>: Use the thumb (and not the middle finger) to sign the number 3.

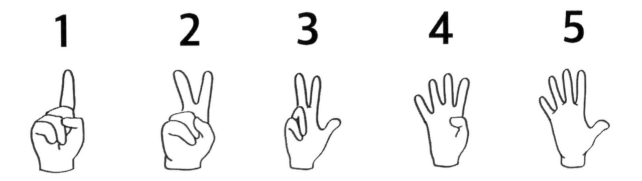

6 to 10

<u>Numbers from 6 to 9 are signed with the palm facing forward.</u>

Look at the picture below so make a circle between the thumb and the pinkie finger for the number 6, and going up to the index finger for the number 9. To sign the number 10 put your thumb up like the "ok" universal gesture and move it back and forth.

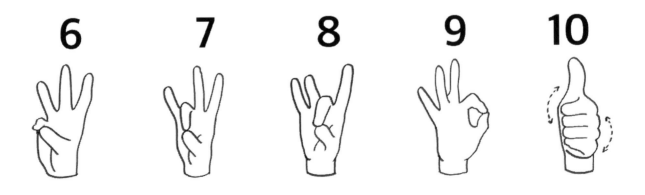

11 to 15

All these signs are made with the palm facing you.
To sign the numbers 11 and 12 you need to flick your fingers up two times starting from the "1" and "2" position. For the numbers 13, 14 and 15 you put your fingers together and pull them in towards yourself.

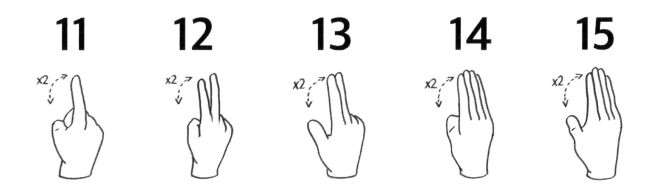

16 to 20

Numbers from 16 to 19 are signed simply twisting twice the second number sign position so 16 is a 6 shacked back and forth and so on. For the number 20 you move from 2 to 0 just tapping your index finger and your thumb together twice.

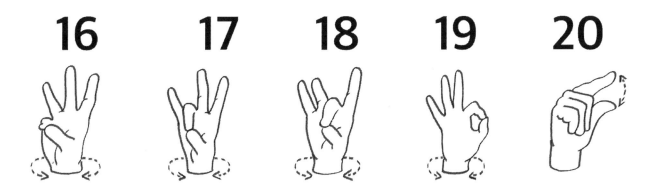

These are the most used numbers. If you want to learn all the others, and find out how to sign a double number and much more, go at the end of the book and scan the QR code for watching the related video!

Days of the week

- **Monday**: Take your "M" and turn it to you making just a little circle.
- **Tuesday**: Take your "T" flipped backwards and moving it in a circular motion.
- **Wednesday**: Take your "W" flipped backwards and moving it in a circular motion.
- **Thursday**: With the palm facing you, move from "T" to "H" pointing your fingers to your non-dominant side
- **Friday**: It's an "F" hand flipped backwards going in the shape of a circle
- **Saturday**: Do the same with your "S" hand
- **Sunday**: Raise your hands with palms facing forward in "5 handshape". Lower them towards your torso, creating a sweeping motion that traces a backward arc from top to bottom.

MONDAY   **TUESDAY**   **WEDNESDAY**

THURSDAY   **FRIDAY**   **SATURDAY**

SUNDAY

Months of the Year

For months composed by five letters or less you have to fingerspell all the letters, but for months that have more than five letters you can abbreviate them fingerspelling just the first three letters.

Here below you can check all the cases:

- **JAN** for January
- **FEB** for February
- **MARCH**
- **APRIL**
- **MAY**
- **JUNE**
- **JULY**
- **AUG** for august
- **SEP** for September
- **OCT** for October
- **NOV** for November
- **DEC** for December

How to sign the Year

As for spoken English you simply divide the year into two parts and you sign them both. So you will sign "19" and "10" for "1910" or "20" and "20" for "2020". Instead for dates that end with a number from 00 to 09 you will sign the first number before, then the double zero just sliding your hand in "0" position and finally the last number.

So now try to sign the dates below:

- January 8, 2003
- April 22, 1996
- September 11, 2001
- December 25, 2023
- Your birthday
- Today's date

Rule of 9

This rule is very important and it explains as we incorporate numbers from 1 to 9 into signs. Here below there are the main examples:
- money
- cents
- age
- time
- hour
- second
- minute
- day
- week
- month
- year

- For "**money**" we have what's called "**the dollar twist**" for all the numbers from 1 to 9. You simply sign the number with the palm facing forward and then quickly twist it moving the palm back. From numbers over 9, you need to sign the number before, and then the "dollar" sign. "**Dollar**" is signed exactly like "**bill**": hold your non-dominant hand open and horizontally before you, palm facing in and thumb sticking up. Then take your dominant hand and use it to grasp your non-dominant hand, starting from the curve at the base of the thumb and sliding to the edge of the index finger. It is like you are tracing the top edge of a dollar bill.

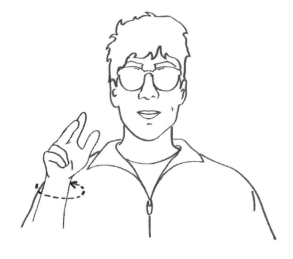

3 dollars

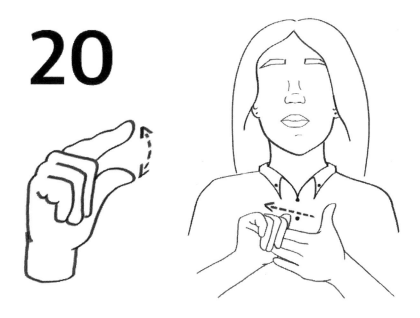

20 dollars

- To sign "**cents**", point your index finger to your forehead while the rest of your dominant hand is held in a fist with palm facing out, then move your hand down at an angle and away from your face. This is also the "**1 cent**" sign so, you incorporate the number in the sign for numbers from 1 to 9. Instead for numbers over 9 you sign "cents" before and then you sign the number.

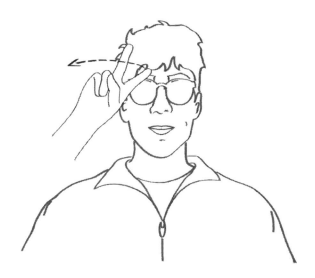

2 cents

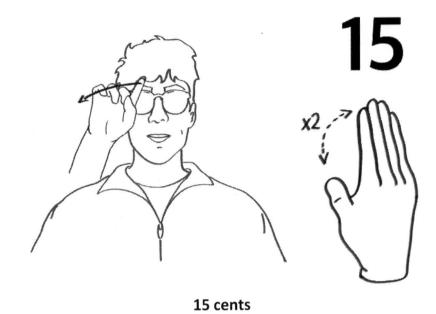

15 cents

For instance, if you want to sign "**3 dollars and 15 cents**" you have to sign:

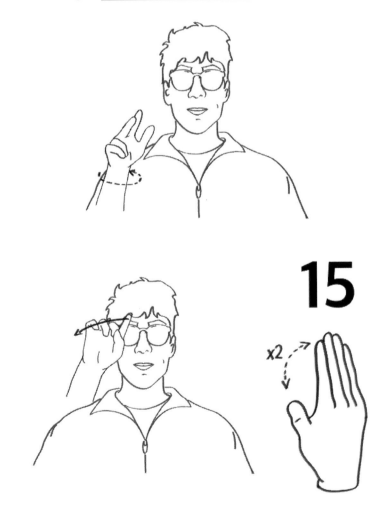

- The sign for "**age**" also can be used to mean "**old**" so, take your dominant hand to your chin while forming the "O "sign. Then pull your hand downward and squeeze the hand closed to end in an S handshape. So, you incorporate the number in the sign for numbers from 1 to 9. Instead for numbers over 9 you sign "age" before, and then you sign the number.

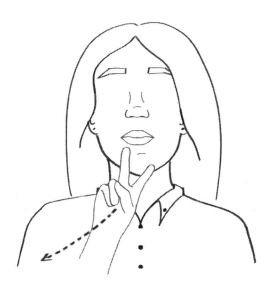

2 years old

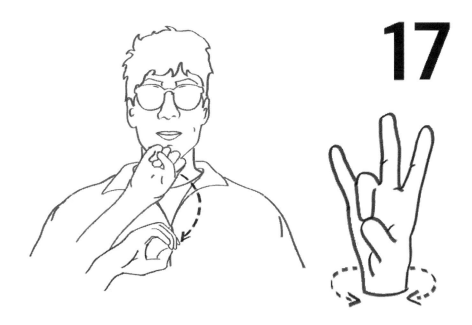

17 years old

- To sign "**time**", we move our dominant hand with the index finger lifted to our wrist and tap twice, as if pointing to a wristwatch. We incorporate the number from 1 to 9 in the sign moving the hand from the wristwatch once. For numbers over 9 we do the same but we start the dynamic part of the sign only when moving the hand away.

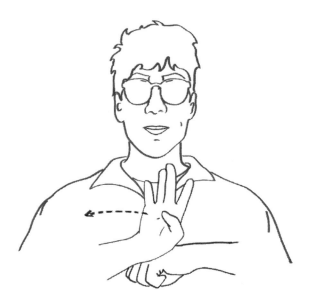

It's 4 o'clock

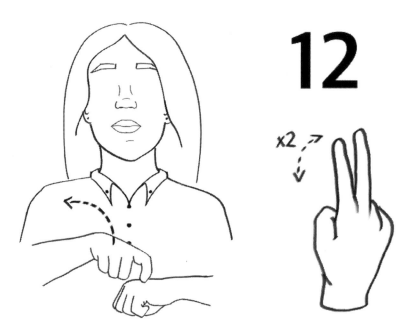

It's 12 o'clock

For instance, if you want to sign "**it's 5 past 4**" is enough to sign the hour before and then you sign the number.

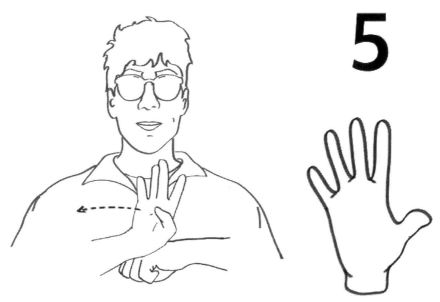

- The sign for "**second**" also can be used to mean "**minute**" (depending on context) and it's generally done on the palm. You "tick" the index finger handshape (of your dominant hand) forward (just moving the wrist and not the finger) as if it were the clock hand on a clock. For the numbers from 1 to 9 you incorporate the number in the sign. For numbers over 9 you sign the number before and then you make the "second" sign with your index finger.

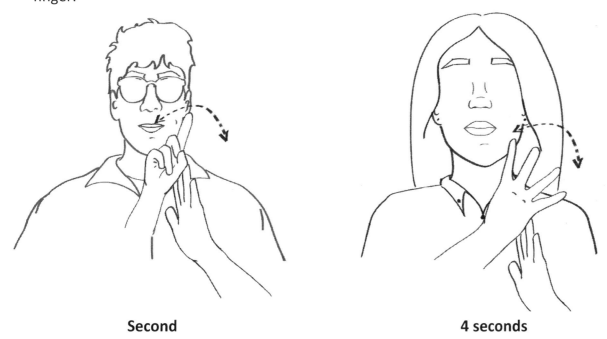

Second   **4 seconds**

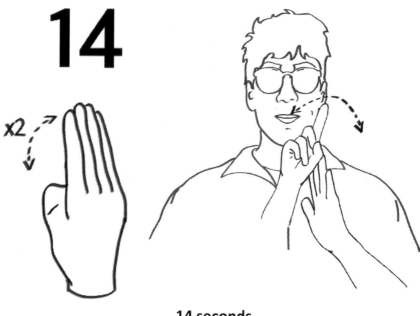

14 seconds

- To sign "**minute**" when you sign from 2 to 9 you point the number to your wrist. For numbers over 9 you sign the number before ant then you make the "minute" sign with your index finger.

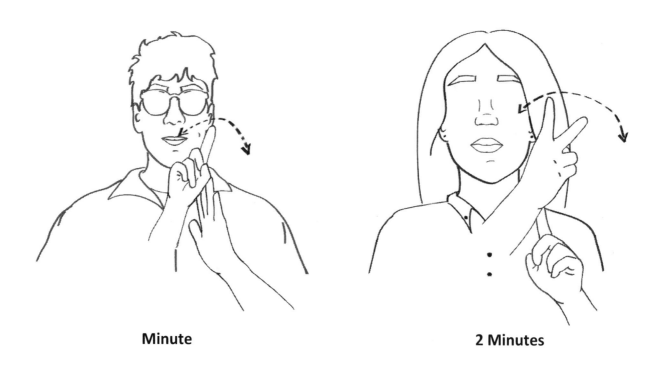

Minute   **2 Minutes**

- To sign "**hour**" you need to represent, with your dominant hand, the movement of the "minute hand" of a clock going around one-time. Instead with the other hand you represent the face of the clock. For the numbers from 1 to 9 we incorporate the number in the sign but for numbers over 9 we sign the number before and then we sign "hour".

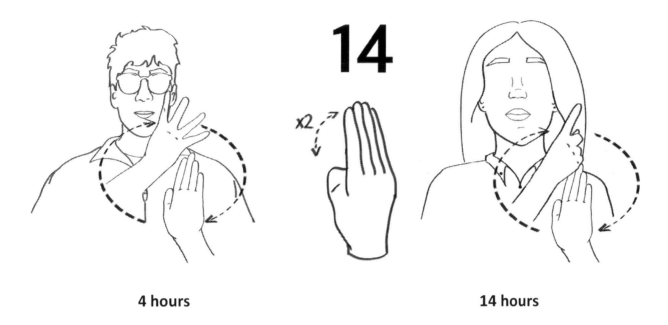

4 hours   **14 hours**

- To sign "**day**" imitate the imagine below: for numbers from 1 to 9 we incorporate the number in the sign but for numbers over 9 we sign the number before and then we sign "day".

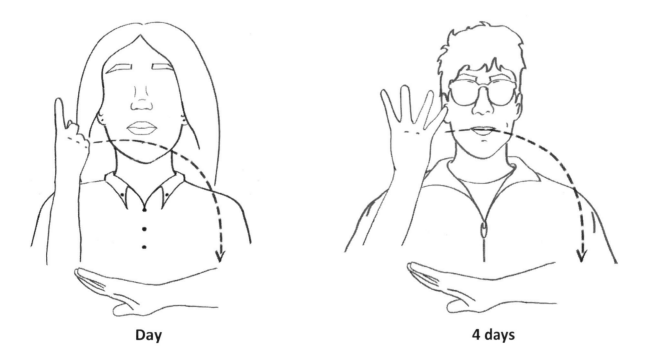

Day   **4 days**

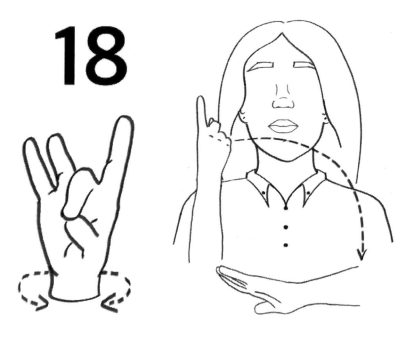

18 days

- To sign "**week**" take your non-dominant hand and hold it out flat, with your palm facing up. Now slide the back of your dominant hand, in fisted position with the index finger raised up, towards the outside of your other hand. For the numbers from 1 to 9 we incorporate the number in the sign but, for numbers over 9, we sign the number before and then we sign "week".

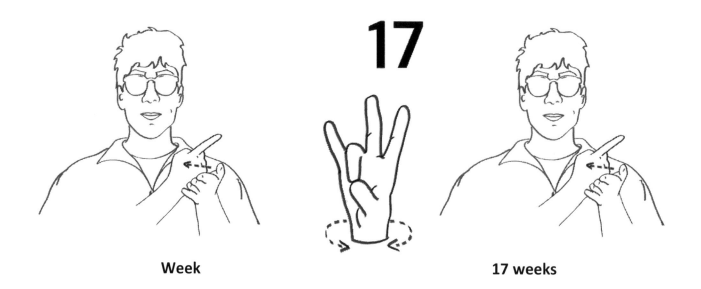

Week   **17 weeks**

- To sign "**month**" keep both your hands in "1" position. So, keep your non-dominant hand in an upright position, place your dominant hand horizontally in front of the other hand and lower it from the top of your non-dominant index finger to the back of your non-dominant hand. For the numbers from 1 to 9 we incorporate the number in the sign but for numbers over 9 we sign the number before and then we sign "month".

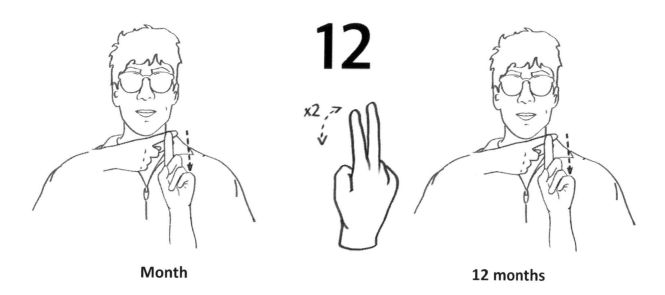

Month   **12 months**

- To sign "**year**" keep both your hands in "S" position. Start with your dominant hand beneath the non-dominant one. Rotate it fully around, concluding the movement with your dominant hand on top. For the numbers from 1 to 9 we incorporate the number in the sign but for numbers over 9 we sign the number before and then we sign "year".

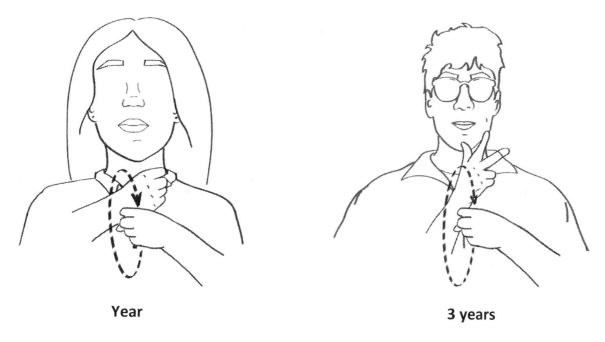

Year   **3 years**

Pronouns

There are two different kinds:

- **Personal pronouns**
- **Possessive pronouns**

*In both cases, for signing plural words you just need to change the hand movement.

- **Personal pronouns** are those that refer to a person. To sign them, keep your dominant hand in the "1" handshape and point to the person being referred to.

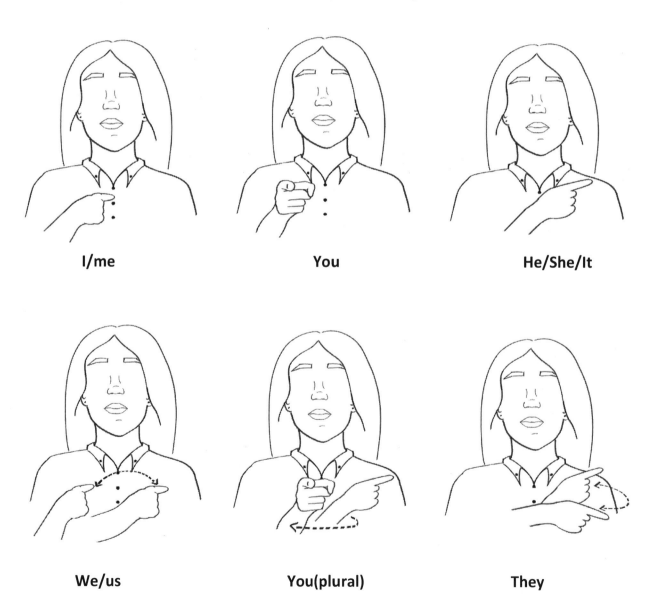

I/me	You	He/She/It

We/us	You(plural)	They

- **Possessive pronouns** instead, are those that refer to things that belong to someone. To sign them, keep your dominant hand in the "open B" handshape and point to the person being referred to.

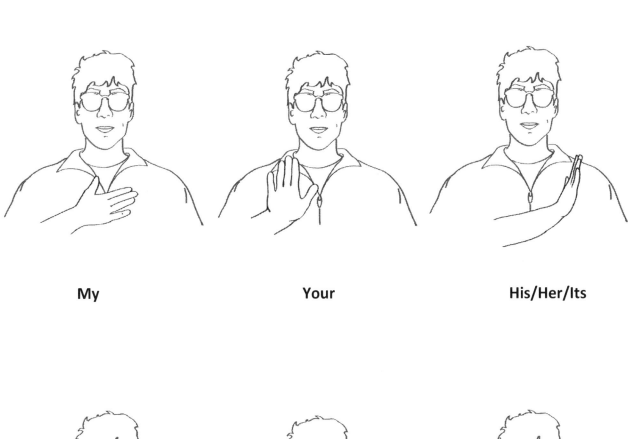

| My | Your | His/Her/Its |

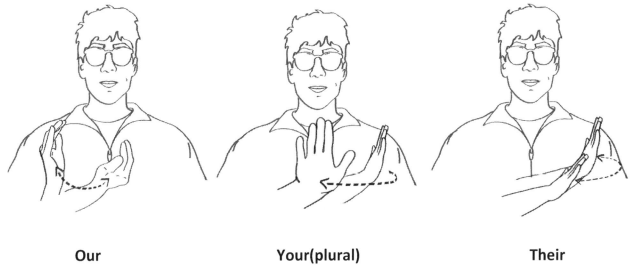

| Our | Your(plural) | Their |

Pluralization in ASL

Pluralization is a process of making a plural of a signed word. In English, you can add "s" to a noun word for plural. Instead in ASL, as we have just learnt for pronouns, a signed word can be modified by a handshape, a movement, a direction, and/or a repetition to signify a degree of plural.

For instance:

- **Child/Children**

"**Child**" is signed by taking your dominant hand with palm facing down and bobbing your hand up and down in front of your body. The sign looks like you are patting a child on the head.

"**Children**" looks like you are patting several children on the head. So, take both hands out in front of you with palms facing down, and bob the hands up and down in front of your body, gradually shifting them outward.

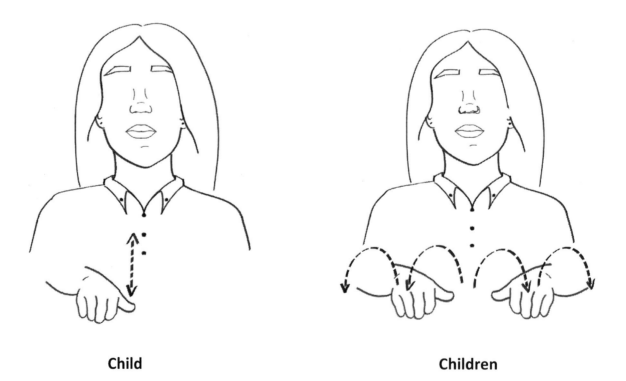

Child   **Children**

Prepositions

Prepositions are words that describe the position of one thing in relation to another.

Instead of static images, I've created a dedicated video to provide a clear and direct understanding of how to sign each preposition.

Additionally, you'll find another video that will guide you through a more in-depth learning experience, incorporating these prepositions into example sentences.
For optimal comprehension, it's recommended to watch this second video towards the end of Book 2, after you've become familiar with phrases.

It's practice time!

Go at the end of the book and scan the <u>QR code</u> for watching the related video and elevate your understanding of these crucial linguistic tools.

<u>In these videos you will learn how to sign:</u>

UP/DOWN: You just point up or down with the index finger.

IN/INTO/INSIDE: You have a cup and you are going to put something into it.

OUT: You have a cup and you are going to pull out something from it.

WHILE/DURING/AS: Point your index fingers out with both palms up, then back towards yourself and at the end roll them under and forward.

SINCE/UP TO NOW: Do the opposite movement, so move your index fingers from the bottom to the top.

ON: Place the open palm of your dominant hand on your non-dominant hand in fisted position.

OFF: Do the opposite movement, so move your dominant open palm outward.

OVER/ABOVE: Rotate in a horizontally circle, your dominant hand, with open palm facing down, above your non-dominant hand in fisted position.

UNDER/BENEATH/BELOW: Rotate in a horizontally circle, your dominant hand, with open palm facing down, below your non-dominant hand in fisted position.

WITH/TOGETHER: Place both your hands together, forming the "A" handshape.

WITHOUT: You do the sign "WITH" and then you just pull both hands apart and open.

THROUGH: You are going to take your dominant hand, facing up, and then put it through the fingers of your other hand.

TO: (the movement from one place **TO** another) Point up the index finger of your non-dominant hand, and tap it with the index finger of your dominant hand.

FROM: hold up the index finger of your non-dominant hand, then use the side of the index finger of your dominant hand to touch the tip of the non-dominant hand's finger. As you do this, pull the dominant hand's finger backwards, turning it into an X shape.

AROUND/ABOUT: Moves the index finger of your dominant hand around and above your non-dominant hand (in "flat 0" position).

BOOK 2:

Greetings and Practical Communication

Book 2 is about to begin, and to ensure you have a solid foundation, make sure you've watched all the related videos. If you haven't already, go to page 101 and scan the QR code.

Basic verbs in ASL

- To sign "**to go**" by pointing with both hands to the direction you wish to go.

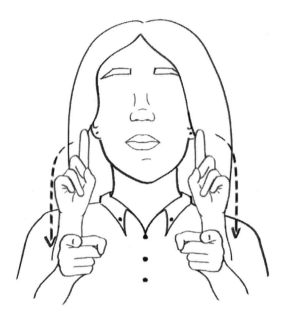

- To sign "**to like**" place your open hand on your chest, pull it away while making your middle finger and your thumb come together ("8" handshape).

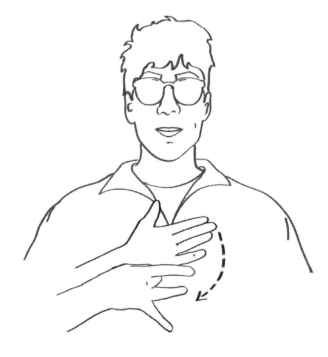

- To sign "**want**", start with both hands opened and facing up and twist them facing down. (Add a negative headshake if you want to make the word negative)

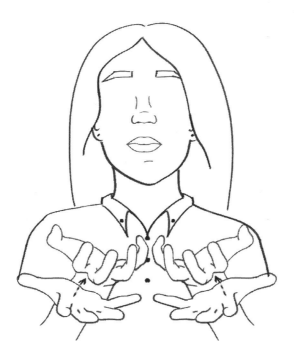

- To sign "**to need**", start from the "x" position and then bend your hand downward from the wrist. (Add a negative headshake if you want to make the word negative)

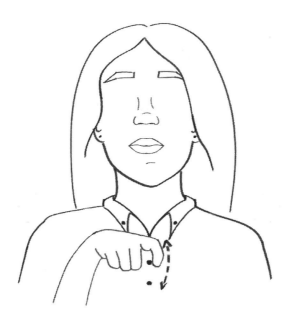

- To sign **"to have"**, hold both hands in "bent" handshapes, and then move them back and touch your chest.

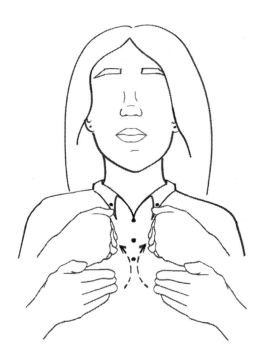

- To sign **"to love"**, place your hands in fisted position and cross your arms across your chest.

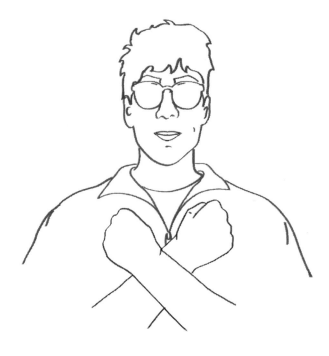

- To sign "**to think**", place your dominant hand in "1" handshape, facing you, and touches the index finger to the forehead.

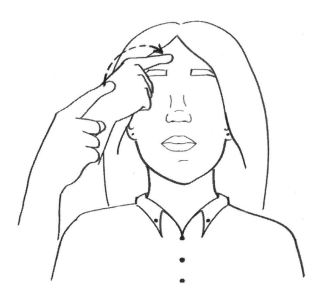

- To sign "**to work**", place both hands in fisted position and use your dominant fist to tap the side of your non-dominant fist twice.

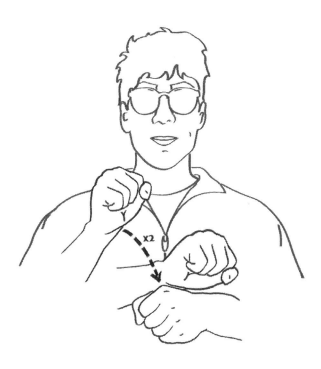

- To sign "**to learn**", place your non-dominant hand with the palm facing up in front of your stomach. Then, use your dominant hand in the "5" position, as if you are attempting to grab something from your other hand.

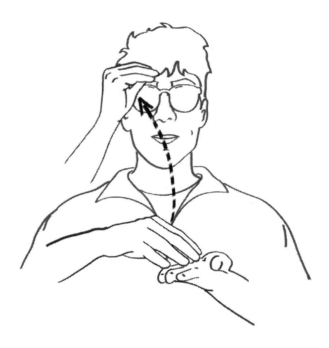

- To sign "**to hear**" (or "**to listen**"), keep your dominant hand in "5" position and point at your ear with your index finger.

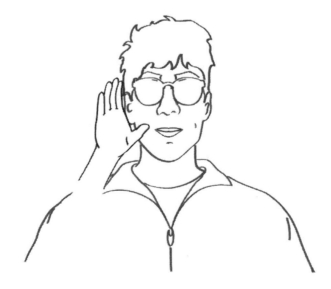

- To sign "**to help**" keep your dominant hand in "A" handshape (with the thumb up), and place it on top of your non-dominant open palm. Then, lift both hands. <u>You can incorporate the subject (me/us/them) in the sign just moving your hands in the right direction</u>.

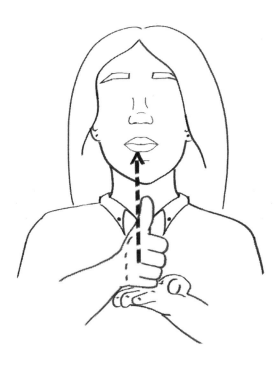

- To sign "**to remember**", make two fists, but extend the thumb out on both. Hold your non-dominant hand steady before you, take your dominant hand's thumb to your forehead and then bring it down to touch your other thumb.

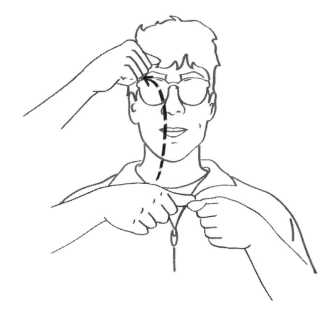

- To sign "**To feel**", keep your dominant hand in "5" handshape and use the middle finger bent at the large knuckle to tap twice on your chest.

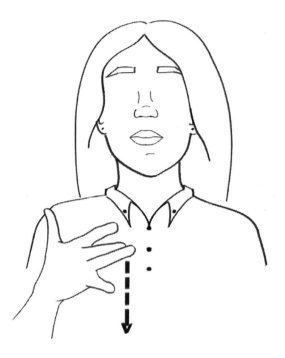

- To sign "**To live**", begin with both hands in a fist position in front of your stomach, then raise them up while tapping your chest with both index fingers.

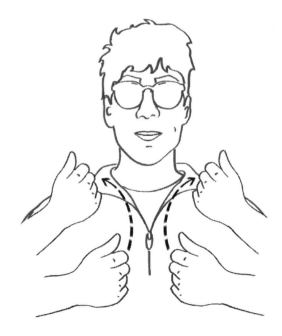

How to build the sentences

In ASL, constructing sentences differs from spoken English. The standard structure is typically Subject-Verb-Object (SVO), but you can rearrange words to emphasize specific elements or better fit the context of the conversation. For instance:

"I love Miami."
In ASL: "MIAMI, I LOVE."

Moreover, non-manual markers play a crucial role in conveying meaning. They can denote exclamatory, negative, or declarative sentences and they are used for punctuation.

*Please note: The "be" verbs (is, are, etc.) are not explicitly used in American Sign Language.

Greetings and basic conversation

So now let's sign how to introduce yourself!

- "Hello, my name is Zac"
- "I am 17 years old"
- "I am from Florida"
- "Nice to meet you"
- "I'm learning ASL"
- "Sign slowly please"
- "See you later"
- "Thank you"
- "Sorry"

- **"Hello, my name is Zach"**

<u>In ASL</u>: Hello-my–name-Z-A-C

To perform the sign "**hello**" simply place your dominant hand (in "open B handshape") with on your forehead close to your ear and move it outwards and away from your body.

To sign "**name**" put your dominant index and middle fingers above your non-dominant index and middle fingers. <u>The facial expression is very important so don't forget to smile!</u>

*At the end fingerspell your name.

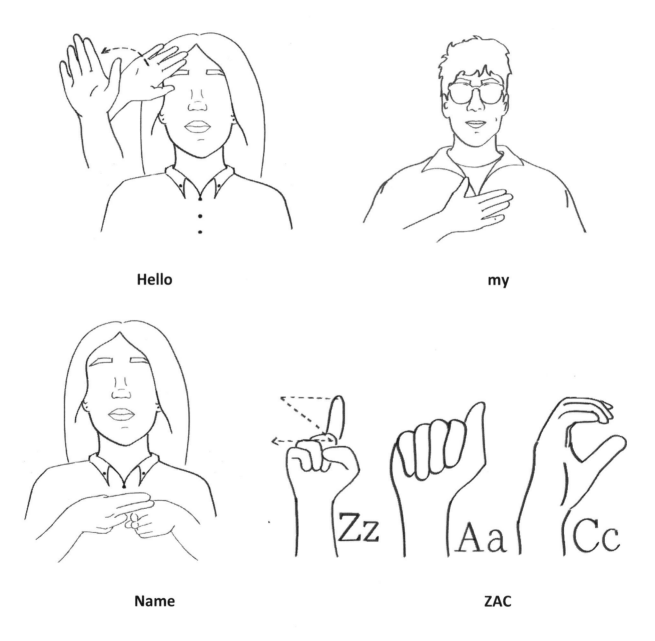

Hello   **my**

Name   **ZAC**

*As you can see, you don't need to put the verb!

- **"I am 17 years old"**

<u>In ASL</u>: me-age-17

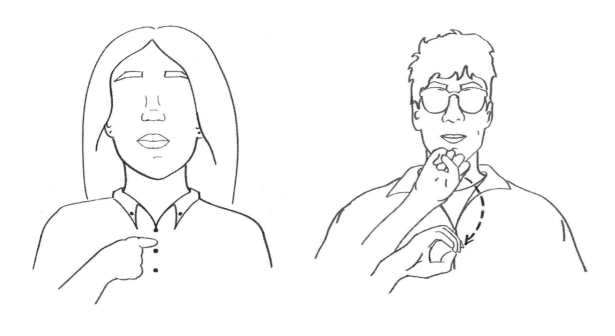

Me   Age

17

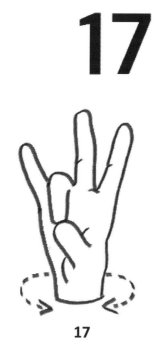

17

- **"I am from Florida"**

<u>In ASL</u>: I-from-F-L-A

To sign **"from"**, hold up the index finger of your non-dominant hand, then use the side of the index finger of your dominant hand to touch the tip of the non-dominant hand's finger. As you do this, pull the dominant hand's finger backwards, turning it into an X shape.

To sign **"Florida"**, you just fingerspell F-L-A.

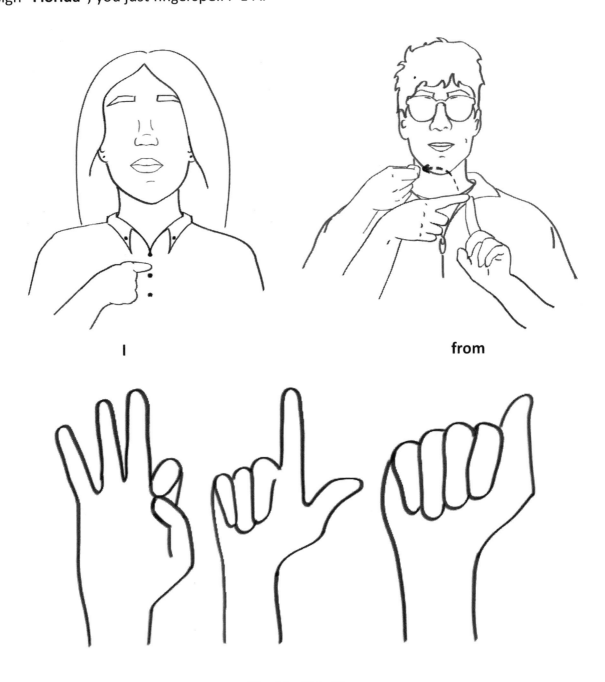

I   from

Florida (F-L-A)

- **"Nice to meet you"**

In <u>ASL</u>: Nice-meet-you

To sign "**nice**" (or "clean"), place your left hand in front of you, palm up and move the flat palm of your right hand across your left hand.

To sign "**to meet**", use "index finger" handshapes. The two hands "meet" in the middle, in front of you. But if you want to sign "**meet you**", you should use the movement direction of the dominant hand to establish who is meeting whom.

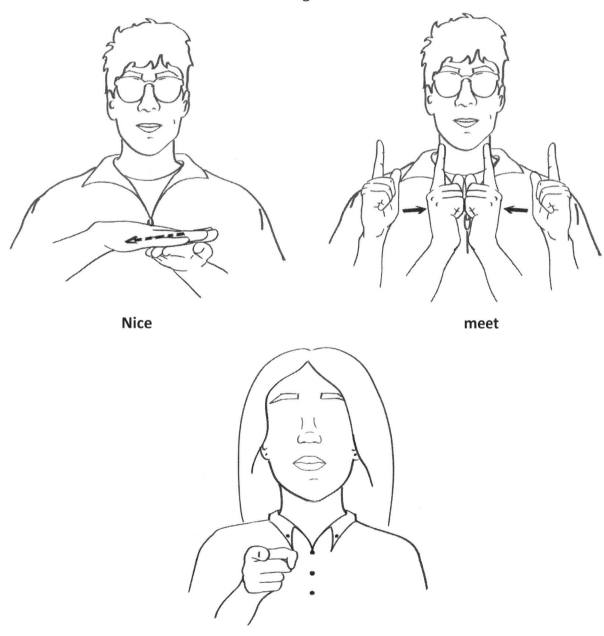

Nice   **meet**

You

- **"I'm learning ASL"**

<u>In ASL</u>: I–learn–A-S-L

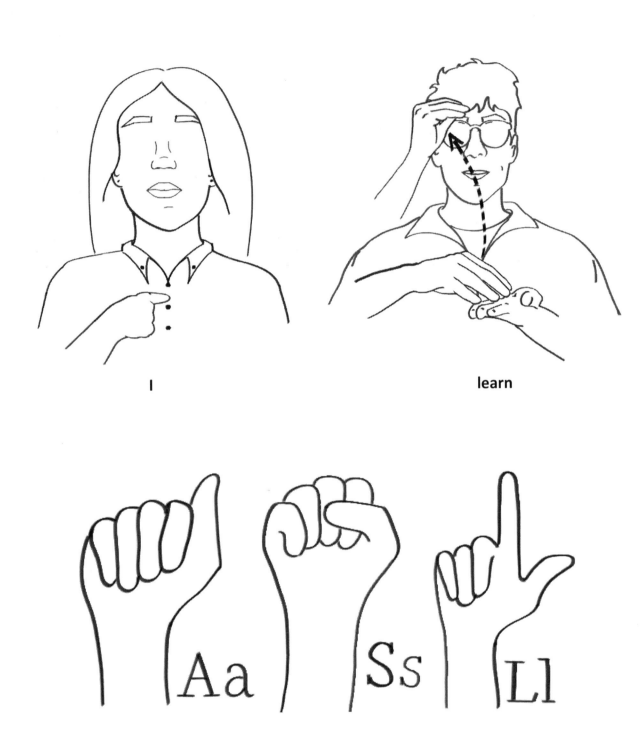

I   learn

Aa   Ss   Ll

- **"Sign slowly please"**

In <u>ASL</u>: sign–slow-please

To sign "**to sign**", place your hands in front of your body in "1" handshape, with the fingers pointing toward one another. Circle your fingers toward your body in an alternating pattern.

To sign "**slow**", slide, just for a few inches, the dominant hand up the non-dominant forearm, beginning at the rear of the non-dominant hand. To sign "**please**", take you dominant hand in "5" position with palm facing in, and rub it in a circle on your chest

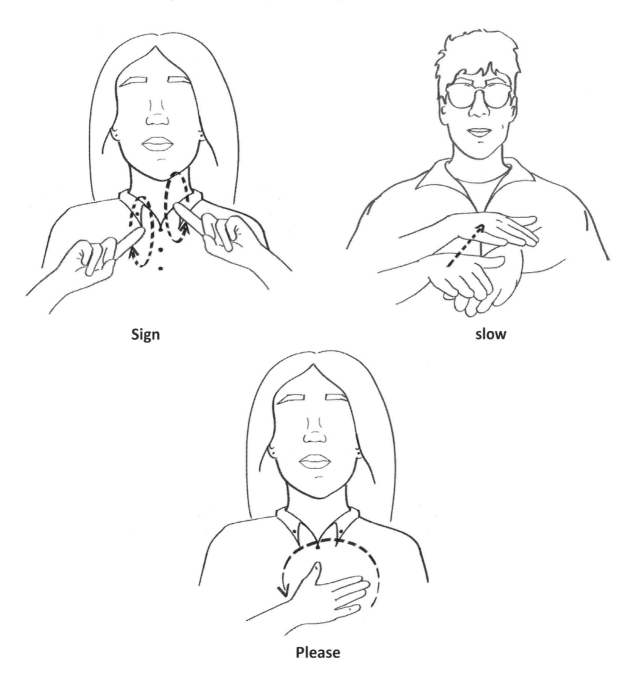

Sign   **slow**

Please

- **"See you later"**

<u>In ASL</u>: See–(you)later

To sign **"to see"**, put your dominant hand in "V" position facing you and move it forward.
To sign **"later"**, take your dominant hand in "L" position palm facing your non-dominant side and turn it down pointing your index finger forward.

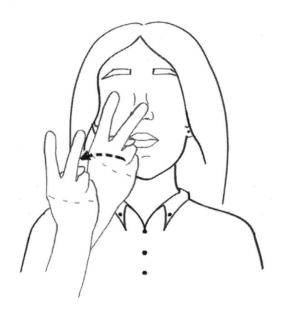

See

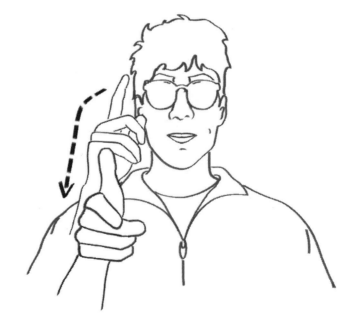

- **"Thank you"**

To sign **"thank you"**, take your dominant hand and touch your fingers to your chin and then bring your fingers forward.

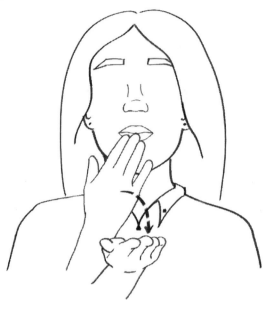

- **"Sorry"**

To sign **"sorry"** make your dominant hand in "A" handshape and rub it in a circular motion across your chest.

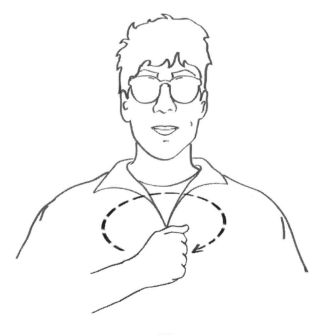

Asking questions

When you want to ask a question, you make a sentence and you add a question word to the end of the sentence. Moreover, you need to use your facial expressions according to the type of the question you are asking.

There are different types of questions but the most used are:

- **"WH" questions**
- **"Yes-no" question**

"WH" questions:

(What, where, who, when, why, which, how)

Your eyebrows are going to go down when associated with that "**Wh**" sentence and also you are going to lean forward when you're signing that.

- To sign **What**, put your hands outwards facing up and shake them back and forth.

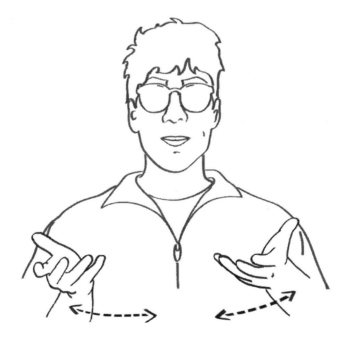

- To sign **Where**, put your dominant hand in "1" handshape and move it from side to side.

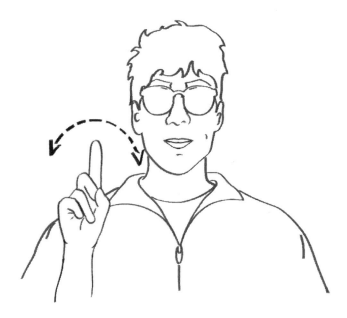

- To sign **Who**, start with a "L" handshape, place your thumb on your chin and bend your index finger twice.

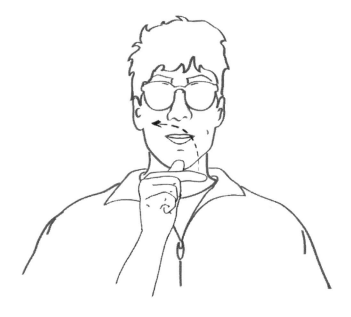

- To sign **When**, put your hands in "1" handshape and twist your dominant hand around to your non-dominant hand, then tap your fingertips together

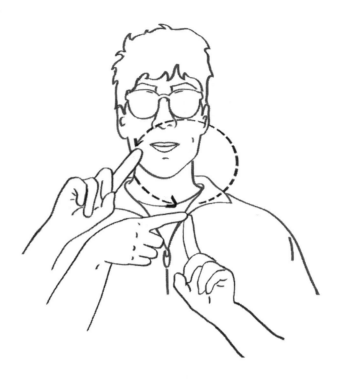

- To sign **Why**, start with your dominant hand facing backward in "5" handshape and move it down while you switch it to a "y" handshape.

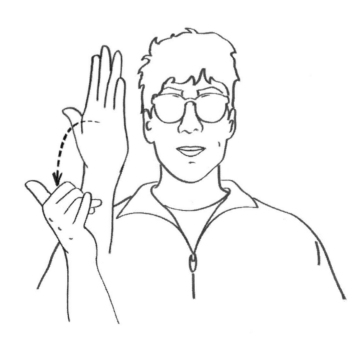

- To sign **Which**, keep your hand facing you in fist position with your thumbs up, and make an alternative movement up and down for two times.

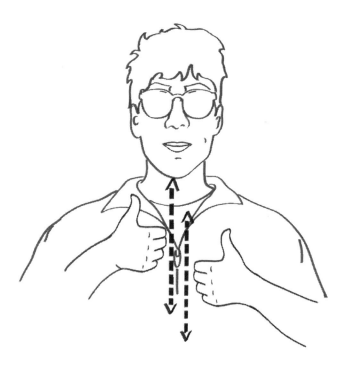

- To sign **How**, keep your hands facing you in fist position with your thumbs up and rotate your dominant hand back and forth while keeping your non-dominant fist steady.

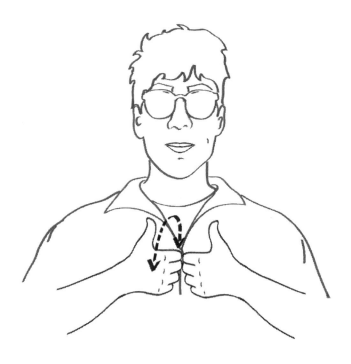

In the next examples you can check how to build a "WH" question. Let's try to sign them!

- **"How are you?"**

In ASL: how-you

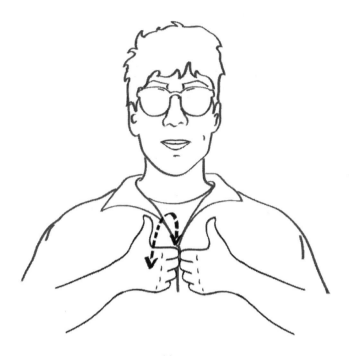

How

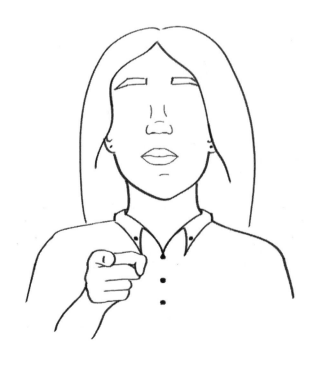

58

- **"Where are you from?"**

<u>In ASL</u>: you-from-where

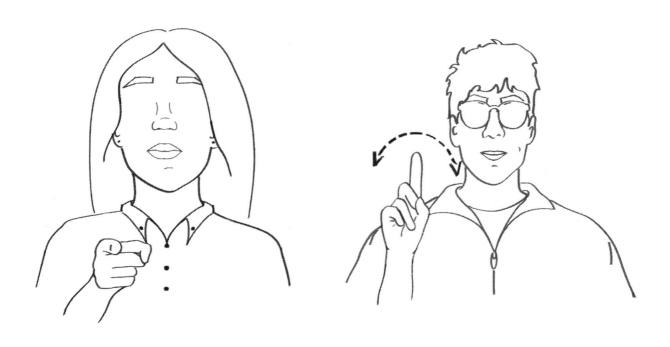

You   **From**

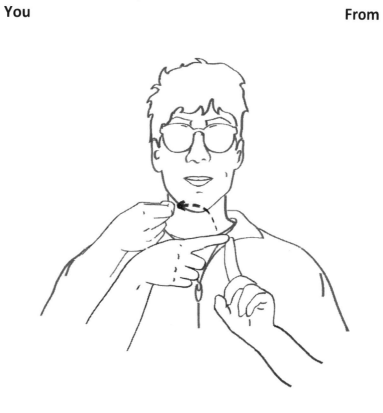

- **"What is your name?"**

<u>In ASL</u>: your-name-what

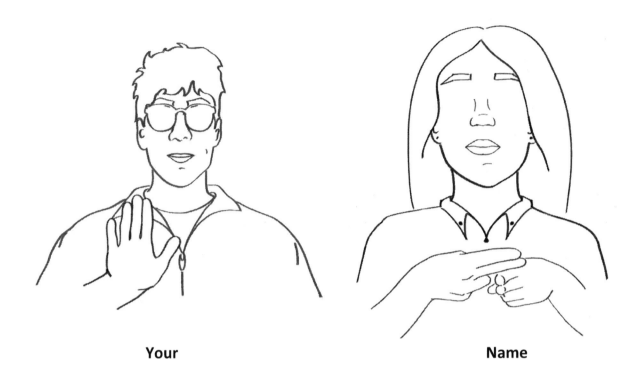

Your   Name

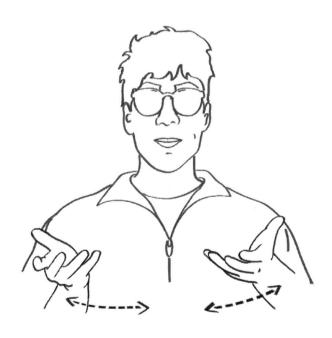

What

- **"Where do you live?"**

<u>In ASL</u>: you-live-where

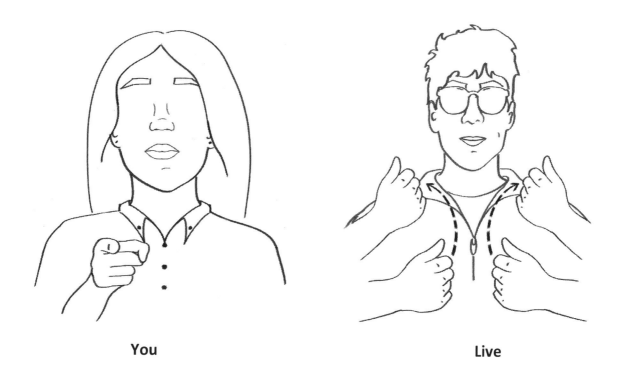

You   Live

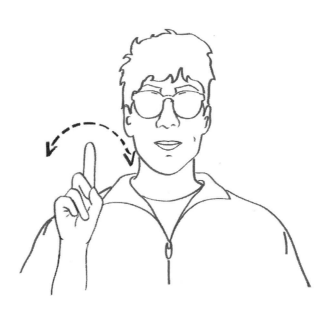

Where

- **"How many brothers do you have"**

<u>In ASL</u>: brothers-you-how many

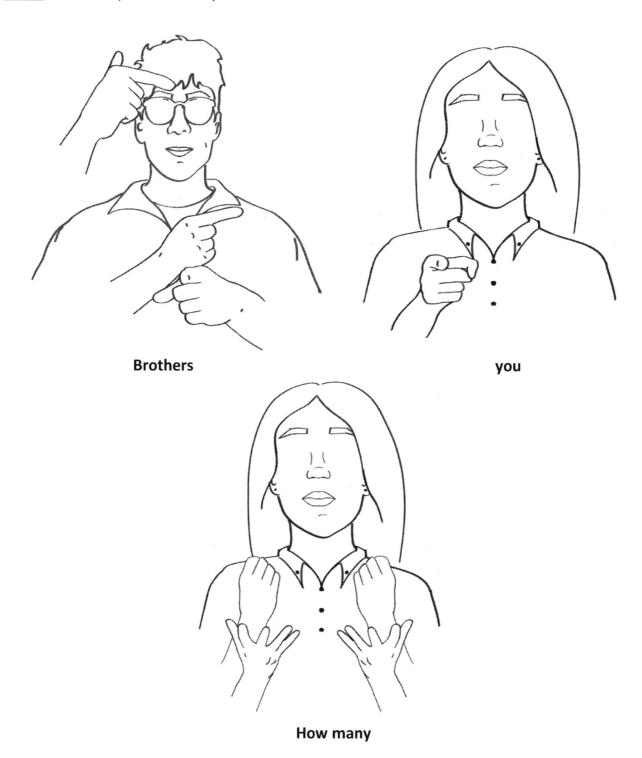

Brothers   **you**

How many

*To sign **"how many"**, begin by forming closed fists, with each hand's four fingers touching the thumb on either side of your body, facing upward. Then, lift your hands upward, keeping your palms facing up and opening your fingers wide.

- **"Where are you learning to sign?"**

<u>In ASL</u>: You-learn-sign-where

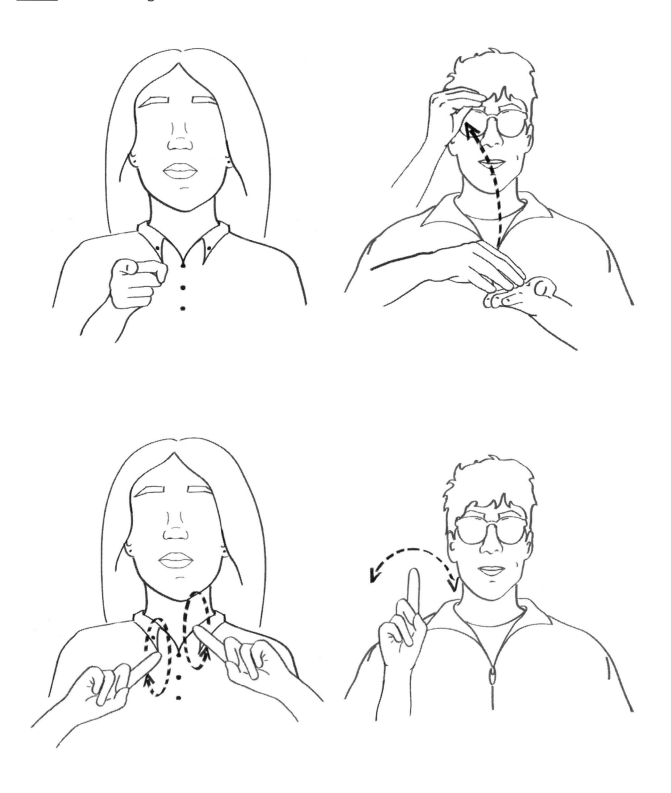

- **"How do you sign the word 'family' ?"**

In ASL: f-a-m-i-l-y-how-sign

First of all, you have to fingerspell the word "family" as we have learnt in the first book.
Then you can sign:

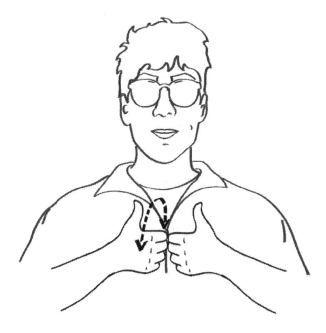

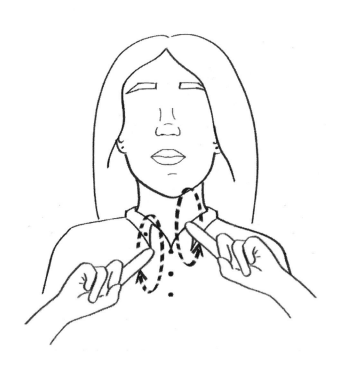

"Yes-no" question

These are the most basic questions and the expected answer is always a YES or a NO. <u>They are normally accompanied by a raising of the eyebrows.</u>

- **"Do you remember...?"**

<u>In ASL</u>: you-remember or remember-you

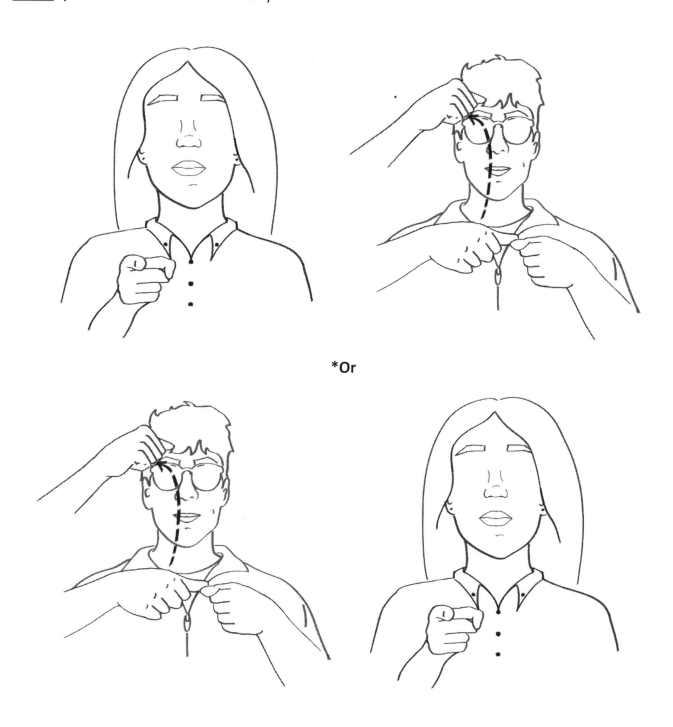

*Or

- **"Are you a hearing person?"**

<u>In ASL</u>: you-hearing

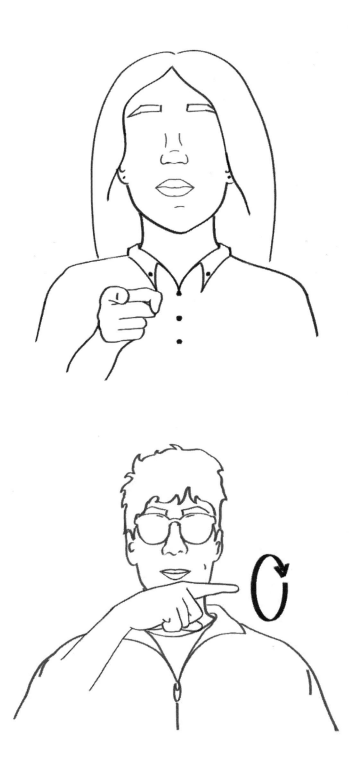

- **"Are you deaf?"**

<u>In ASL</u>: deaf-you

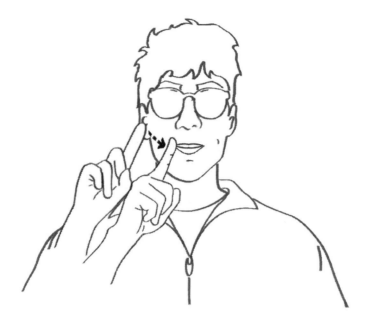

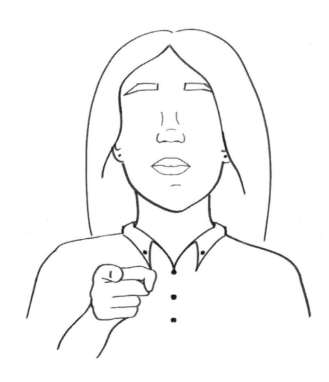

- **"Do you understand me?"**

<u>In ASL</u>: you-understand-me

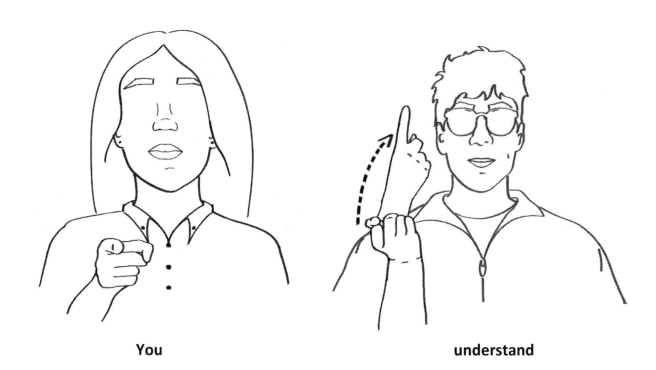

You   **understand**

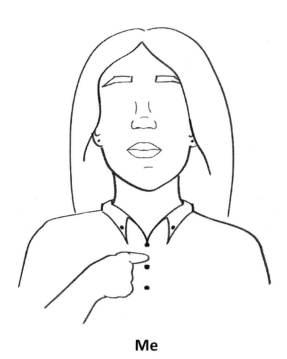

Me

- **"Do you want help?"**

<u>In ASL</u>: you-help-want

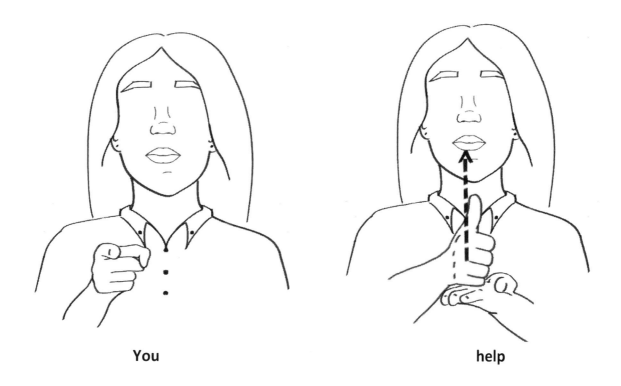

You   help

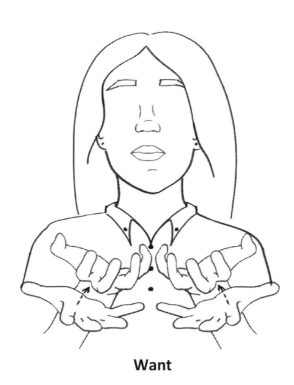

Want

- **"Do you need help learning sign language?"**

<u>In ASL</u>: Learn-sign-need-help-you

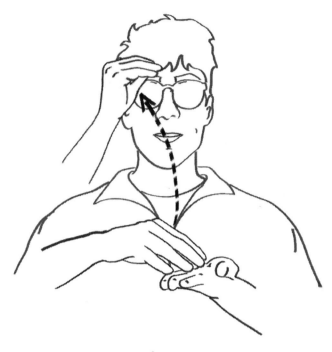

Learn

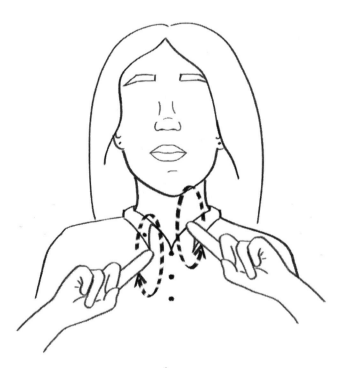

sign

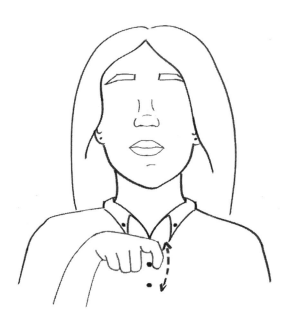

Need

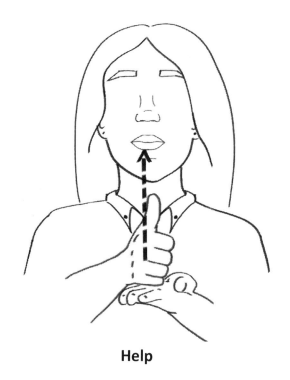

Help

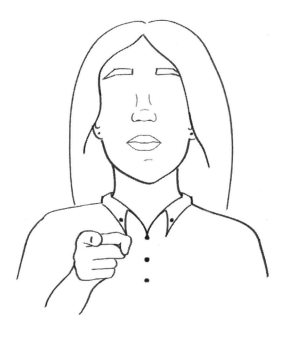

71

- **"Do you have children?"**

<u>In ASL</u>: children-you

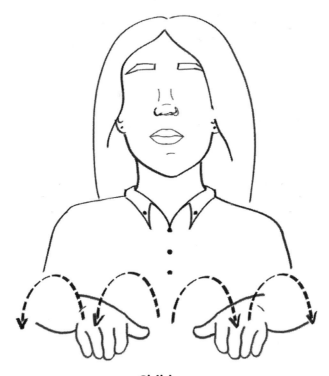

Children

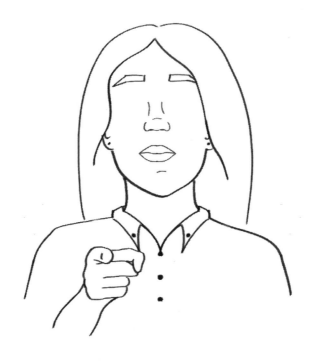

- **"Is your mom deaf?"**

< />In ASL: Your-mom-deaf

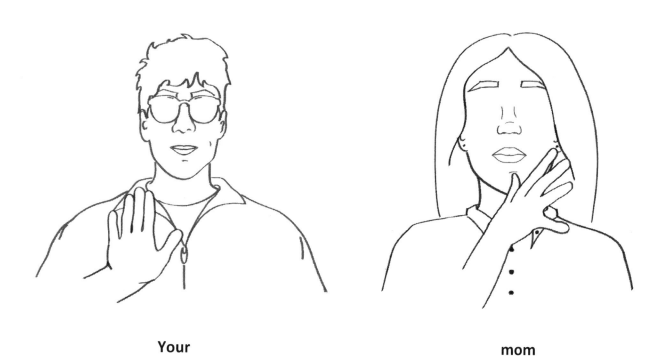

Your   **mom**

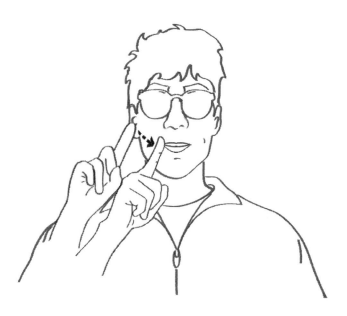

BOOK 3:

Tenses and verb conjugations

It's practice time!

Go at the end of the book and scan the <u>QR code</u> to access all the related videos.

This will enhance your learning experience as you practice with a variety of sentences!

Bodyline system

In American Sign Language, the communication of the verb tenses is not done through verb conjugations as in spoken languages. Instead, ASL utilizes a spatial reference system, named **"bodyline"**, to indicate the timing of an action, whether it's in the present, past or future.

Imagine a line extending in front of you, representing the timeline of an event. When signing a verb slightly in front of your body, you convey the action is in the future. If you sign closer to your body, it indicates the present. Conversely, signing behind your body suggests the action took place in the past.

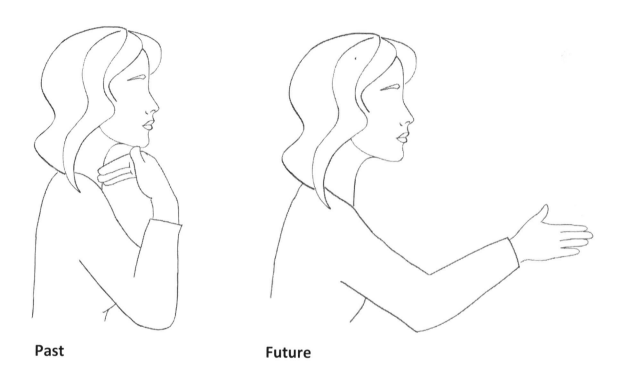

Past   **Future**

So, in ASL, it's not about changing the form of the verb but rather about placing it in the right spot along the "bodyline" to convey the intended time reference.

American Sign Language follows the TIME–TOPIC-COMMENT structure so, when you have an ASL sentence, you're going to put the time at the beginning. If a time is not indicated, then it's assumed to be in the present tense

- **"I am going to the gym"**
  <u>In ASL</u>: future-gym-I-go

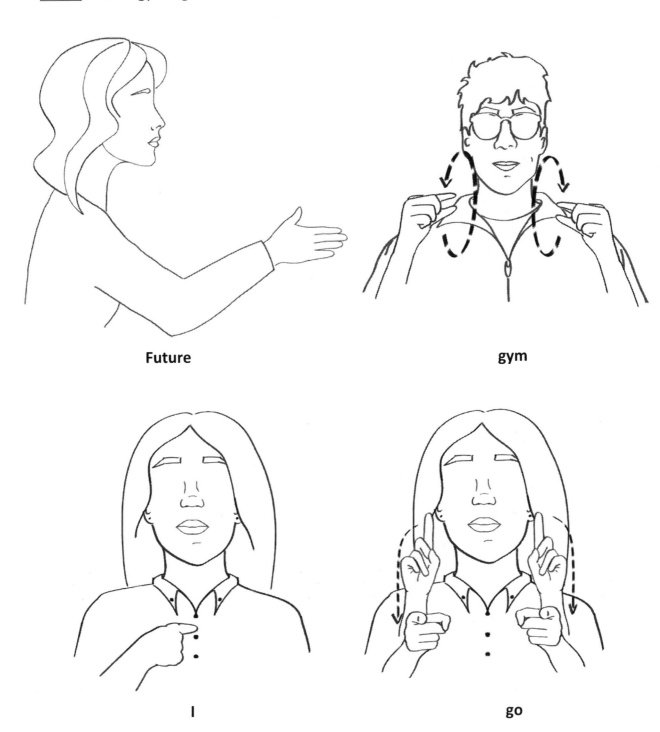

Future   gym

I   go

- **I went to the gym**
  <u>In ASL</u>: past-gym-I-go

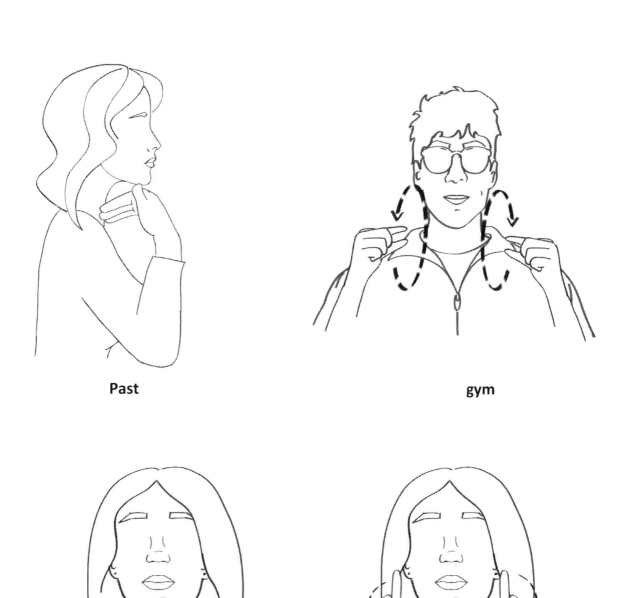

Past   gym

I   go

Here below you can check how to sign the most used temporal signs:

- Today, tomorrow, yesterday;

If you want to learn all the temporal signs, go at the end of the book and scan the QR code for watching the related video. You will learn how to sign:

- in few days, next week, next month, next year;
- recently, few days ago, last week, last month, last year.

- To sign "**today**" place both hands in "Y" handshape in front of your chest, then move them at your stomach level. This sign is also used to sign "**now**".

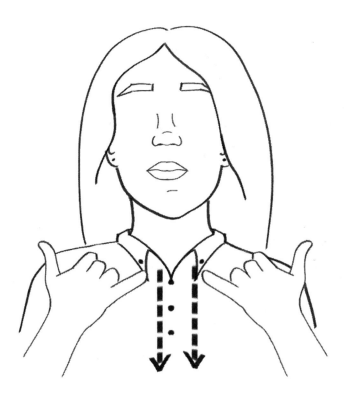

- To sign "**tomorrow**" form a "open A" handshape with your dominant hand, touch your thumb to your chin and then move it forward, away from your face.

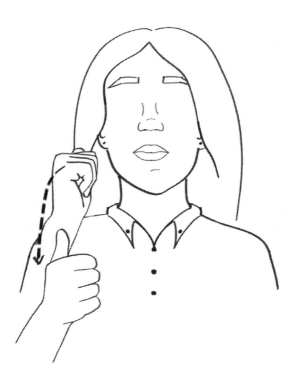

- To sign "**yesterday**" form a "open A" handshape with your dominant hand, touch your thumb to the side of your chin and then move it backward to touch your jawbone.

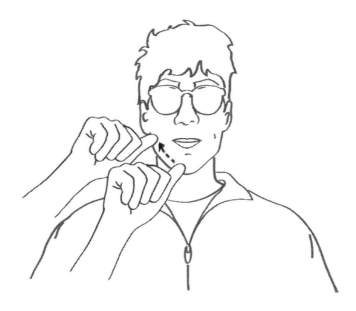

Feelings and emotions

When you sign the emotions, make sure that your hand gestures are matched by your facial expressions!

- **Happy**: Keep both hands flat on your chest and move them up.

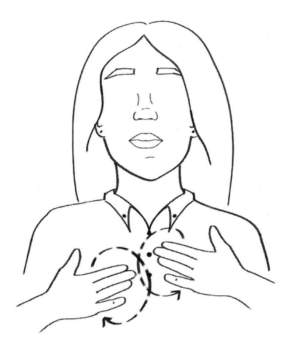

- **Sad**: Place both hands in front of your face with the palms facing you. Bring them down the length of your face.

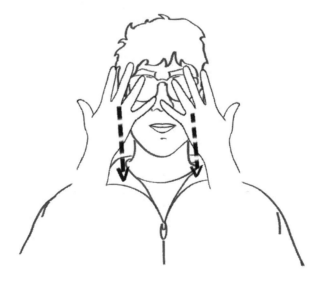

- **Nervous**: Put both hands in front of you facing down and shake them as if you are nervous and you can't keep your hands still.

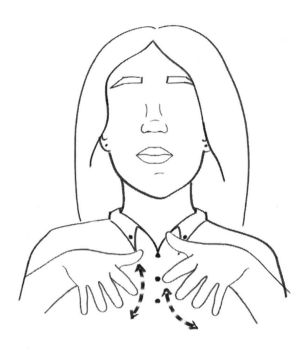

- **Afraid/scared**: Both your hands are coming into your body like you're really scared of something.

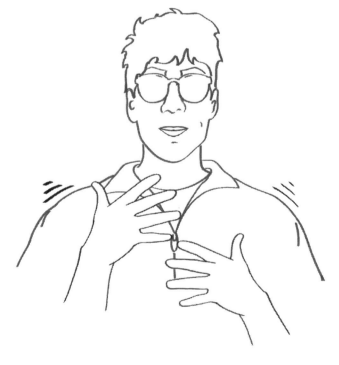

So, now let's try to sign some complete sentences about emotions!

- "Today I'm feeling really sad".
- "What scares you?"
- "I am so nervous for the test tomorrow."
- "I'm happy."

- **"Today I'm feeling really sad".**

<u>In ASL</u>: today-me-feel-sad

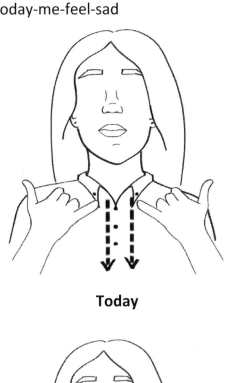

Today

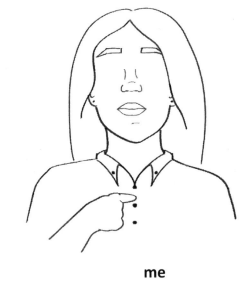

me

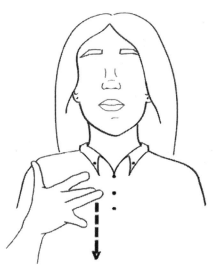

Feel

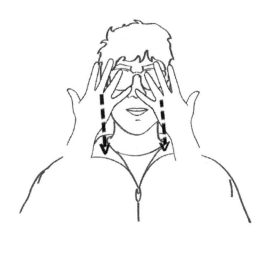

sad

- **"What scares you?"**
<u>In ASL</u>: you-afraid-what

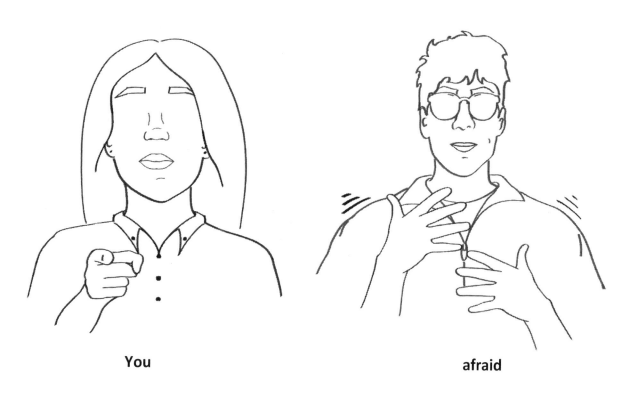

You   afraid

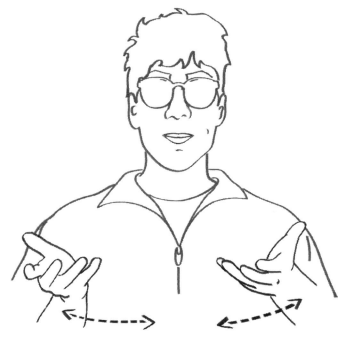

- **"I am so nervous for the test tomorrow."**

<u>In ASL</u>: Test-tomorrow-me-nervous

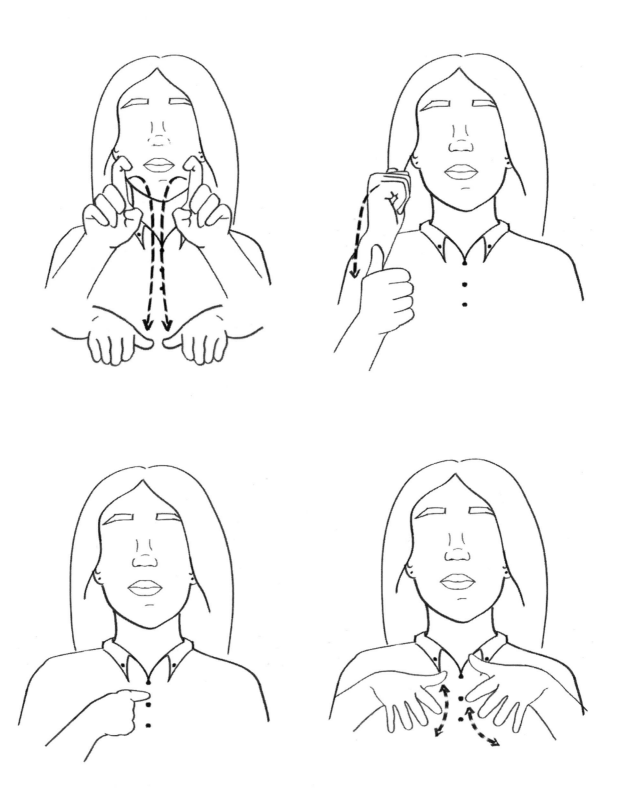

- **"I'm happy."**

In <u>ASL</u>: me-happy

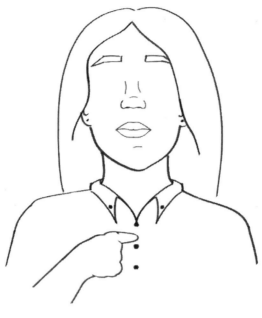

Me

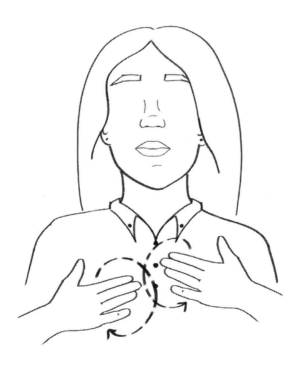

happy

Differences between ICONIC and ARBITRARY signs:

Iconic signs are gonna be signs that look like what they represent

Es: "banana"

This is an iconic sign because it looks like you're peeling a banana.

So, form the "1" hand shape with your non-dominant hand facing towards you. Simultaneously, your dominant hand "is peeling away the banana's skin".

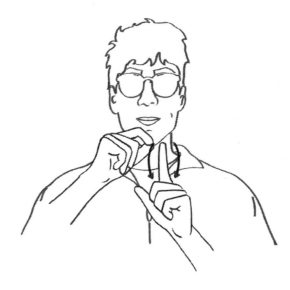

Arbitrary signs are signs that do not look like what they represent

Es: "Apple"

To sign "apple," close your hand and place the knuckle of your dominant index finger against your cheek while simultaneously pivoting your hand back and forth.

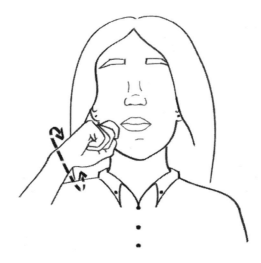

Additional Vocabulary

- To sign "**boy**", put your dominant hand in front of your forehead and tap your index finger and other fingers together.

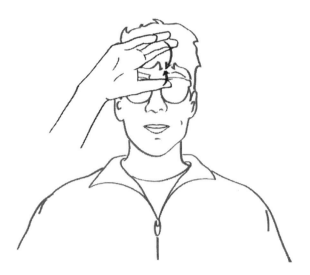

- To sign "**girl**", start by forming a fist with your thumb raised. Then, bring your hand to your face and slide your thumb down your cheek twice.

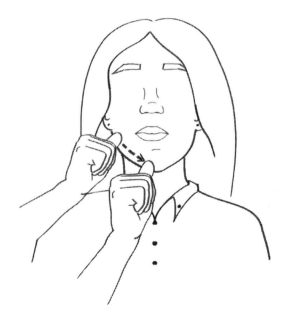

- To sign "**home**", bring your fingers and thumb together and touch your cheek near the side of your mouth. Then move your hand toward your ear and touch your cheek again.

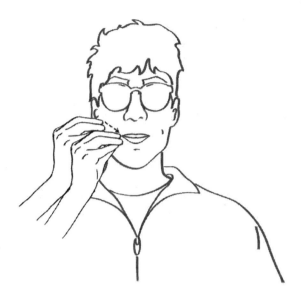

- To sign "**family**", put both hands in "F" position in front of your torso with the two "F" touching at the index fingers and thumbs, then forming a circle with both hands horizontally.

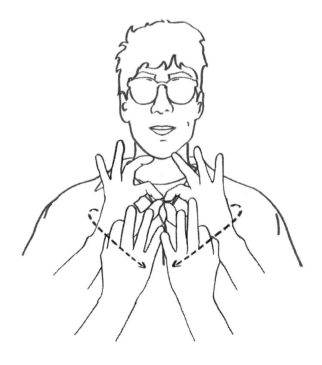

Family – Vocabulary

- To sign "**MOM**", point your thumb at your chin.

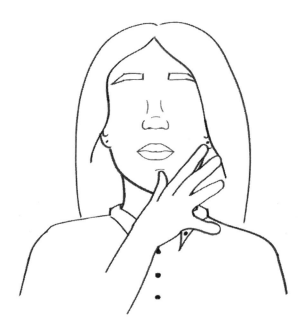

- Instead to sign "**DAD**" point your thumb at your forehead.

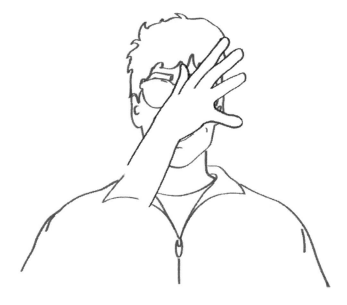

- To sign "**brother**", put both hands in "L" shape with your index and your thumb extended. The non-dominant "L" hand should be by your chest pointing outwards as you are pointing a gun. Instead, your dominant "L" hand should be on your forehead with the thumb and the index finger touching the forehead. Then bring it down to rest on your left hand as a double "L".

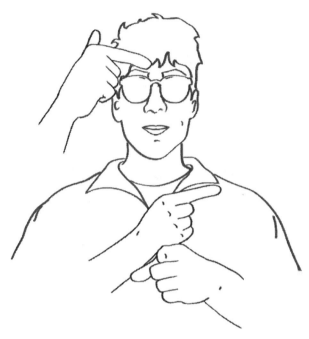

- To sign "**sister**", put both hands in "L" shape as before but move your dominant hand starting from your jaw (and not from your forehead).

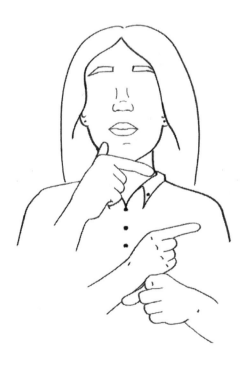

If you want to learn all the signs about "family", go at the end of the book and scan the QR code for watching the related video. You will learn how to sign:

- home, family, friend, boy, girl, dad, mum, brother, sister, cousin, uncle, aunt, grandma, grandpa, husband, wife and son.

Time to Apply Your Knowledge

Now that we've covered some vocabulary related to 'family', it's time to put your knowledge into practice. Let's engage in a series of sentences that encapsulate everything you've learned so far:

- **"I have one brother and two sisters"**
<u>In ASL</u>: 1-brother-2-sisters-I-have

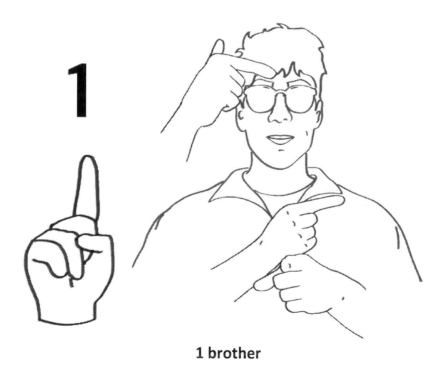

1 brother

2

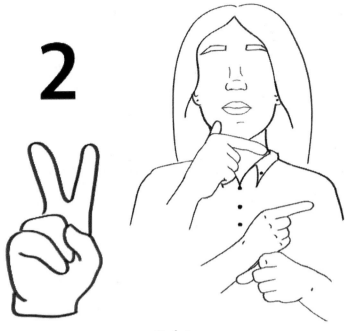

2 sisters

I

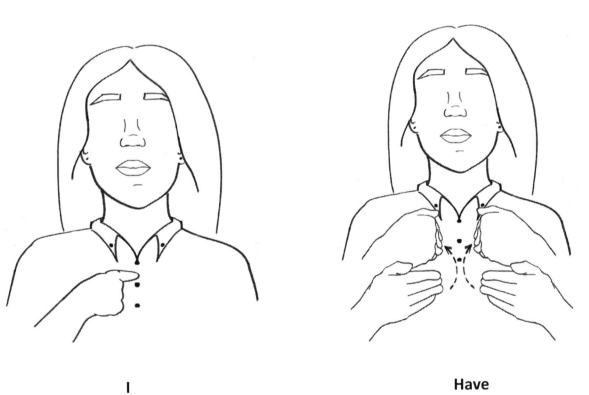

Have

- **"My mum has 2 sisters"**

<u>In ASL</u>: 2-sisters-my-mum-has

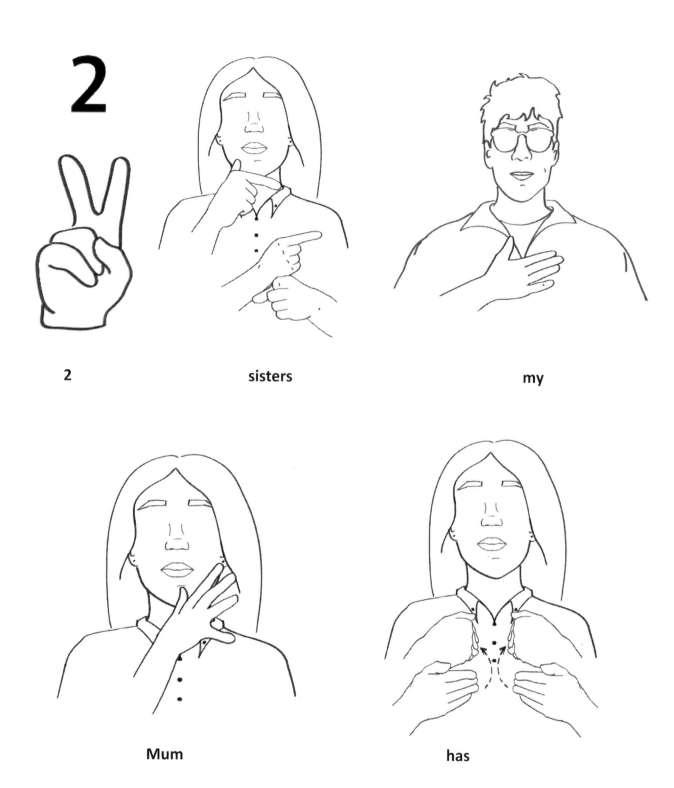

| 2 | sisters | my |

| Mum | has |

- **"Do you want to go home now?"**

<u>In ASL</u>: you-want-go-home-now

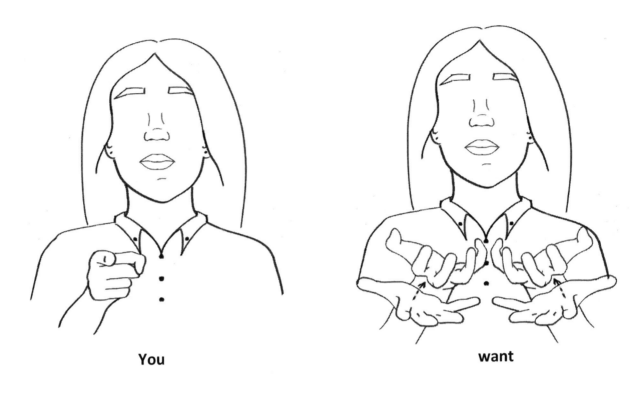

You
want

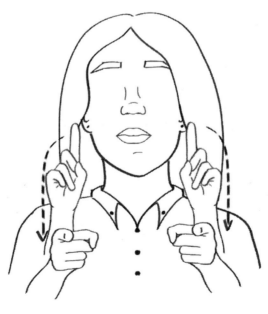

go

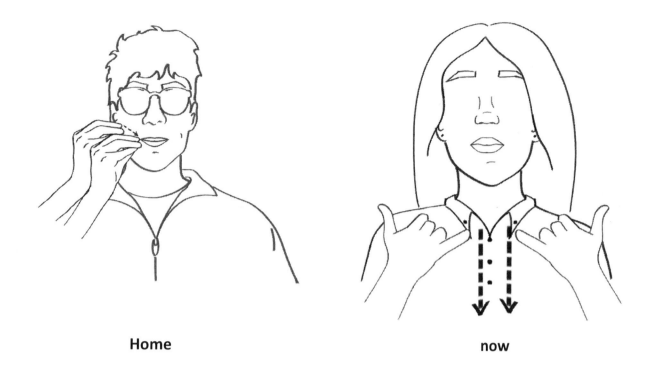

Home   now

- **"Is his brother going to school tomorrow?"**
In ASL: tomorrow-his-brother-go-school

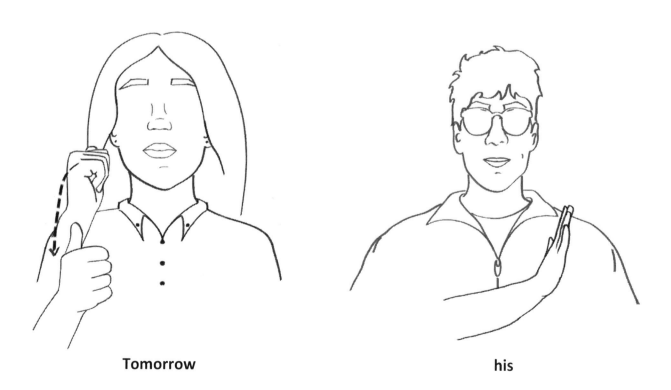

Tomorrow   his

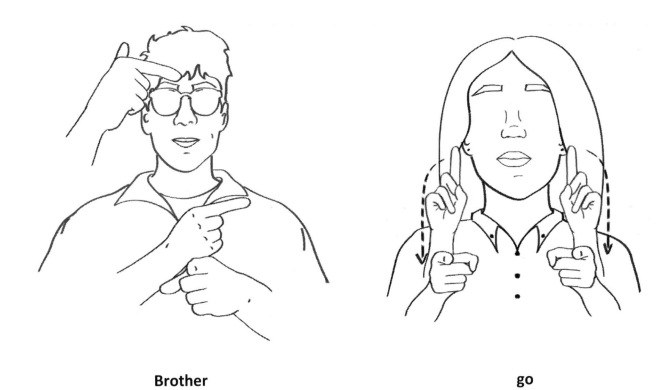

Brother   **go**

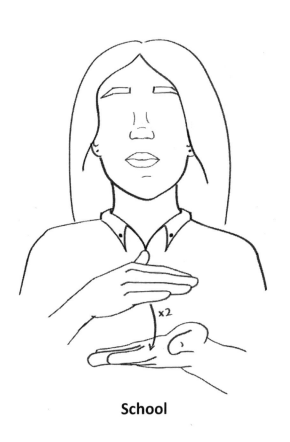

School

- **"What is your dad's name?"**

<u>In ASL</u>: Your-dad-what-name

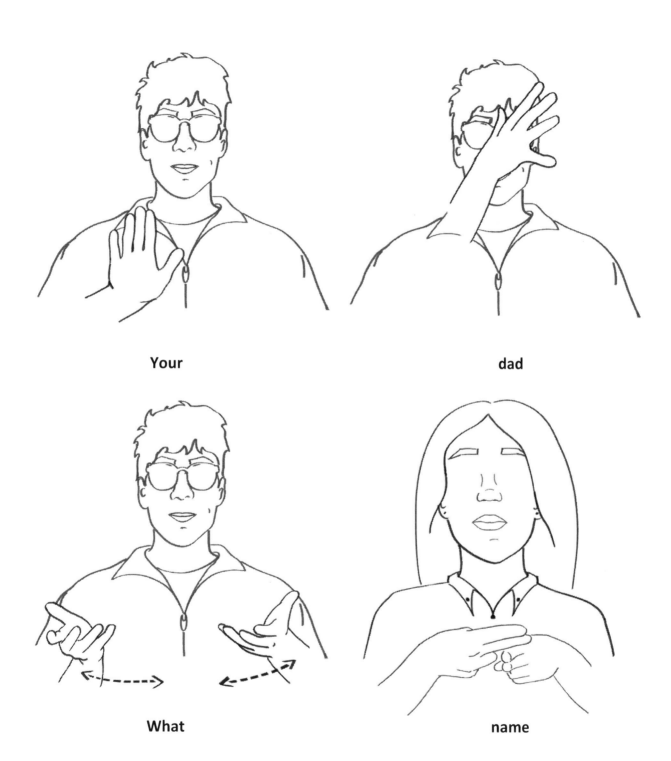

Your

dad

What

name

- **"Do you like your work?"**

<u>In ASL</u>: You-like-your-work

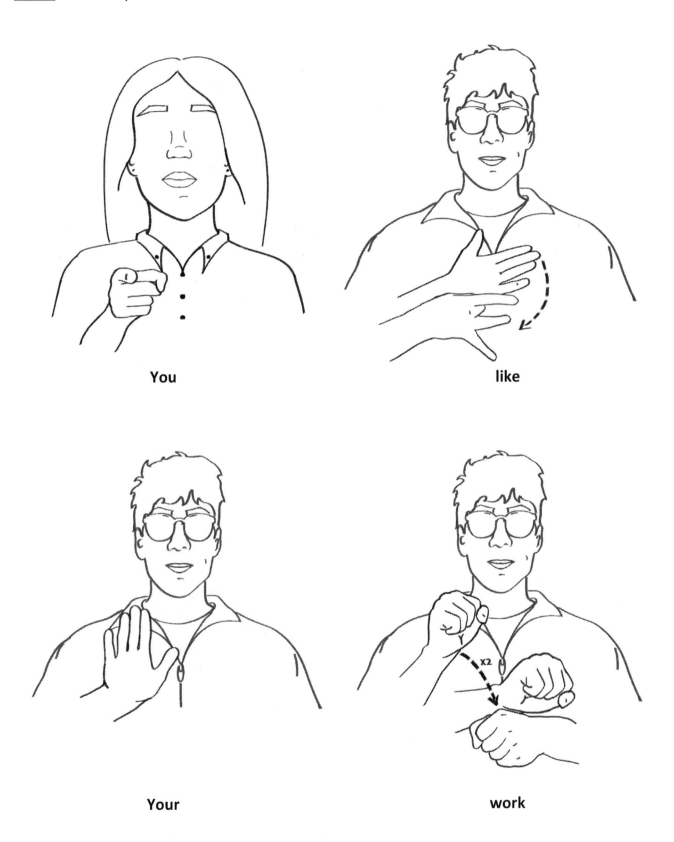

You

like

Your

work

- **"Do you think I sign good?"**

In ASL: You-think-I-sign-good

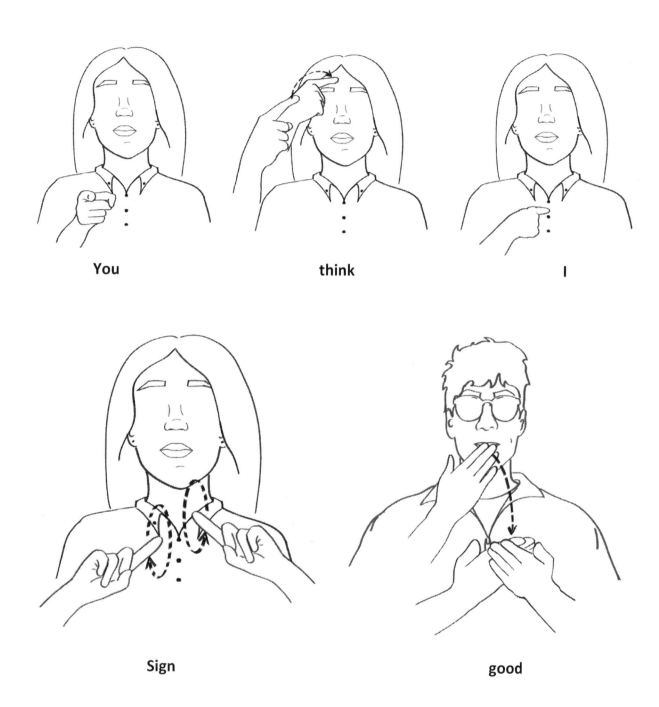

You	think	I

Sign	good

To sign "**good**", start with your dominant hand in "open b" handshape at your mouth and move it into the palm of your left hand. Both hands should be facing upward.

Conclusion

In this journey through American Sign Language (ASL), you have acquired the fundamental basics of a unique and fascinating language. Now, you possess the ability to communicate, connect, and understand a community that utilizes this rich and vibrant form of expression.

Remember that your learning doesn't end here. ASL is a continuous journey of discovery and deepening. I encourage you to keep practicing, exploring, and sharing your knowledge with others. Every sign you make is a step toward more inclusive communication and deeper understanding.

Thanks for selecting this book to accompany you on your learning adventure. I hope your knowledge of ASL not only enriches your life but also contributes to making our world a more inclusive place for everyone.

A sincere thanks to Daisy, our extraordinary collaborator, and to you, the reader, for your commitment to learning and sharing sign language. Your contribution represents a crucial move towards a world where communication is accessible to all, overcoming hearing barriers.

I really would like to hear your thoughts about your experience because your input is valuable and can inspire those who want to start this rewarding journey.

How about suggesting new signs or topics you'd like to learn? Leave your request in a review, and I'll do my best to quickly add new video lessons on what you want to learn!

Scan the QR code below to access an entire collection of bonus tutorial videos.

"Thank you for choosing my book.
Your review on Amazon would be greatly appreciated and supportive."

Made in the USA
Columbia, SC
07 December 2024

48643707R00057